Heal
DEFENCE
Cookbook

Portia Spooner
and
Dr Paul Clayton

Photography by **Johnny Boylan**
and **Belinda Pickering**

Food stylist: **Sonja Edridge**

Edited by Joanna Downs

© Accelerated Learning Systems Ltd, Aylesbury, Bucks, UK

First published 2001 by Accelerated Learning Systems Ltd
Tel. 01296 631177 www.acceleratedlearning.com

ISBN 0 905553 65 9

DR PAUL CLAYTON SAYS

The media may like to talk about the impact of genes on our health – because that's news. But it is still true that what we eat is, along with exercise, the most important influence on whether we live out a full and healthy life.

Long term studies show very large differences in the incidence of disease in different populations. For example, the incidence of breast and prostate cancer and heart disease in Japan and Korea is much lower than in Europe or the USA. Specific items in their diet have now been identified – such as soy products – which confer considerable protection against these diseases.

Based upon these sorts of studies plus large-scale nutritional trials, it is now possible to list many of the nutrients that confer the highest levels of protection against degenerative disease. That is the theme of the recently published book *Health Defence*.

This is its companion – a cookery book that enables you to boost your intake of the most protective nutrients that science has identified – but through recipes that are totally in tune with the British palate.

That's where the art of the cook meets the science of nutritionist. I have been extremely fortunate to be able to team up with TV chef Portia Spooner. She has taken my list of desirable ingredients and turned them into delicious, and above all, practical meals that will grace any table. If you combine the advice in this cookbook with the advice in *Health Defence*, you and your family will become 'global eaters' – taking the best from every culture's diet. And your nutritional intake would put you in the top 1% of healthy diets on the planet! Enjoy!

Paul Clayton

How to use this book

We start with a glossary of selected foods, showing why they are well worth emphasising in your cooking. The notes on Page 8 explain some of the less familiar terms.

At the end of each recipe DR CLAYTON SAYS: summarises the benefits from the main ingredients in it, and one or more symbols show the potential of those ingredients to reduce your risk of a major health threat. The more often a symbol is repeated, the stronger the protection.

Obviously one meal has little impact – the real value lies in building up a repertoire of recipes that, used consistently, will have a long-term effect on your health and longevity.

 heart disease
 bowel problems
 joint damage
 osteoporosis

 deteriorating brain function
 skin ageing
 eyesight degeneration

Look for more recipes on **www.healthdefence.com**.

This lists by category the main foods used in this book and their health benefits. The categories are: Eggs, Fish, Fruit, Grains and flour products, Herbs and spices, Milk and dairy products, Nuts, Vegetables and Miscellaneous.

Eggs

Eggs contain lecithin phospholipids which increase levels of HDL cholesterol (the 'good' cholesterol). They also contain carotenoids and the more intensely coloured the yolk, the higher the carotenoid content; free range eggs contain higher levels of these valuable micro-nutrients. Carotenoids have anti-cancer properties and protect the eyes and skin.

Fish

Herring are an excellent source of Omega 3 Polyunsaturated Fatty Acids (PUFAs), which have strong cardio-protective properties. PUFAs have also been shown to reduce inflammation of the airways and joints, and can help to reduce the symptoms of asthma and arthritis. Herrings also contain iodine (essential for thyroid function); traces of selenium; and a useful combination of calcium and Vitamin D which can help to maintain healthy bones.

Mackerel: similar to herring

Salmon: similar to herring. Wild salmon are preferable to farmed, as they generally contain significantly higher levels of the valuable and cardio-protective Omega 3 PUFAs. They also typically contain higher levels of astaxanthin, a carotenoid with anti-oxidant and anti-cancer properties.

Sardines contain some Omega 3 PUFAs, also calcium and Vitamin D, and traces also of iodine.

Shrimps/prawns (especially fresh water) contain betaine which can reduce blood levels of the toxic compound homocysteine, thereby reducing the risk of heart attacks. Betaine is also found in squid, mussels, oysters, sugar beet and spinach, but is most easily consumed in supplement form.

Fruit

Apples contain the flavonoid quercitin, which is anti-oxidant and probably cardio-protective, Vitamin C and fibre (pectin) which lowers blood cholesterol levels, if consumed in sufficient amounts.

Apricots are a good source of beta carotene and fibre, and also flavonoids.

Avocados provide a mix of mono-unsaturated and poly-unsaturated fatty acids (MUFAs and PUFAs) which are cardio-protective. They also contain B vitamins and Vitamin E.

Bananas: an excellent source of complex carbohydrates, and pre-biotics, as we s being rich in potassium (which may reduce blood pressure) and dietary

Blackberries: similar to blackcurran

Blackcurrants contain high level Vitamin C and flavonoids linked increased protection against heart disease, various cancer nd the loss of vision that can con pa abetes.

Blueberries: simil

Cherries (es similar to black

The health benefits of selected foods

Citrus fruit (oranges, lemons, grapefruit, etc) contain Vitamin C and flavonoids with many therapeutic properties. They are anti-inflammatory, cardio-protective and probably have anti-cancer properties.

Dried fruit: in general, a good source of dietary fibre and flavonoids.

Mangoes are an excellent source of beta carotene, plus Vitamin C and dietary fibre.

Pears contain Vitamin C, dietary fibre and traces of B vitamins and some minerals. Perhaps their most interesting ingredient is the polysaccharides which form the gritty particles in pear skin. These are immuno-stimulants, similar to those found in shiitake mushrooms (see below).

Prunes have high levels of flavonoids, and may also contain pre-biotic compounds as well as dietary fibre.

Raisins are similar to red wine without the alcohol, but contain more sugar! A good source of flavonoids. Currants are particularly good, sultanas less so. (Their lighter colour indicates a lower level of flavonoids.)

Raspberries: similar to blackcurrants, although not quite as good a source of flavonoids.

Redcurrants: similar to raspberries. Blackcurrants contain far higher levels of the valuable flavonoids – as evidenced by their darker colour.

Strawberries contain Vitamin C and some flavonoids.

Tomatoes and tomato products are the rich source of lycopene, a carotenoid strong cardio-protective and anti-cancer properties.

Grains and flour products

Bread is a source of B vitamins, calcium and magnesium. It also provides dietary fibre. **Wholemeal breads** tend to provide more of these micro-nutrients than white breads. **Granary bread** is a rich source of dietary fibre. It contains rather more iron and zinc than white bread and also contains B and E vitamins.

Brown rice provides dietary fibre, and a range of B vitamins. Nutritionally superior to white rice, which has a higher glycemic index (see notes), brown rice also has a more interesting texture.

Bulghur wheat: similar to brown rice.

Couscous: similar to brown rice.

Oats are a good source of dietary fibre, and have been shown to lower blood cholesterol levels. They contain beta glucans, an excellent pre-biotic that protects the lower bowel and liver, together with B vitamins, some Vitamin E and various minerals including traces of chromium.

Pasta is a good source of carbohydrate with a medium glycemic index.

Sushi rice: rice bran contains interesting actives which lower blood pressure and induce a calming effect. See also brown rice.

Wheatgerm: traditionally one of the best sources of Vitamin E.

Herbs and spices

Black pepper contains a combination of pepper oils and flavonoids which have been shown to protect against ageing of the brain.

Cayenne pepper has trace pepper oils, with anti-oxidant properties.

Cinnamon is claimed to increase the activity of insulin, and to be of some use in Type 2 diabetes, but this has yet to be substantiated.

Coriander is reported to have anti-oxidant and digestive properties.

Cumin is reported to have anti-oxidant and digestive properties.

Ginger provides ginger flavonoids which have marked anti-inflammatory properties and are also probably cardio-protective.

Mustard contains sulphur compounds that boost synthesis of protective enzymes in the body.

Oregano (marjoram) is a rich source of flavonoids, powerful anti-oxidants with marked anti-inflammatory and anti-ageing properties; capable of stimulating the body's own detoxifying enzyme defences.

Paprika: a powdered extract of peppers (see under vegetables/peppers).

Parsley has some diuretic effect, if consumed in large amounts. It contains various anti-oxidants.

Thyme: similar to oregano.

Turmeric provides a group of flavonoids called curcuminoids, which have many therapeutic properties. They include anti-inflammatory, cardio-protective, anti-diabetic and anti-cancer activities.

Milk and dairy products

Cheeses contain varying amounts of salt, which can contribute to increased blood pressure. They provide calcium and magnesium, but tend to be high in saturated fat.

Crème fraiche (preferably low fat) is a good source of calcium, needed for growing healthy bones and teeth.

Fromage frais has some protein and traces of B vitamins.

Milk (preferably skimmed milk for adults): similar to crème fraiche.

Quark: see fromage frais.

Yoghurt: natural live yoghurts contain pro-biotic bacterial species. Not all are effective, but some may protect against gastro-intestinal infections.

Nuts

Almonds contain MUFAs and Omega 6 PUFAs, as well as Vitamin E, which may help to prevent heart disease.

Brazil nuts contain MUFAs and Omega 6 PUFAs which may help to prevent heart disease. They also provide Vitamin E, which is additionally cardio-protective, and high levels of selenium, a mineral with powerful anti-cancer properties.

Pecans: a nut containing MUFAs, Omega 6 PUFAs and Vitamin E.

Pine nuts contain MUFAs, Omega 6 PUFAs, Vitamin E and flavonoids.

Pistachio nuts have traces of MUFAs, Omega 6 PUFAs, Vitamin E and flavonoids.

Walnuts contain MUFAs, Omega 3 and 6 PUFAs and ellagic acid, which are thought to be cardio-protective, as is their Vitamin E.

The health benefits of selected foods

Vegetables

Artichokes (globe) are a useful source of fibre.

Artichokes (Jerusalem) are an excellent source of inulin, a pre-biotic fibre which protects the lower bowel, the liver and the heart.

Beansprouts are a good source of B vitamins and dietary fibre, with some Vitamin C.

Beetroot contain a group of flavonoids, which give them their intense red/purple colour, the most prevalent of which is called betalain. This flavonoid is not thought to be particularly therapeutic, however, as it is unstable.

Black-eye beans (or black beans) are a good source of fibre. They also contain B vitamins, and are an excellent source of carbohydrates with a low glycemic index (see Notes). They may also help to lower blood cholesterol levels.

Broccoli is an excellent source of Vitamin K, essential for healthy bones; sulphur compounds linked to cancer protection; the anti-oxidant Vitamin C; lutein, which protects the eyes, and dietary fibre.

Carrots contain, as the name implies, beta carotene. Darker red carrots contain higher levels of this micro-nutrient, and are one lucky enough to be able to buy West Indian carrots (which are almost purple in colour) is getting maximum carotenoids and taste! Carrots also provide dietary fibre, and some Vitamin C.

Celery contains compounds that lower blood pressure (if eaten in large quantities), also fibre and traces of B vitamins.

Chillies provide flavonoids, and capsaicins, which create the sensation of 'hotness'. They trigger histamine release, which may make them troublesome for asthmatics.

Chives: similar to onions.

Courgettes have traces of B vitamins and minerals.

Cucumber contains traces of B vitamins and trace minerals.

Garlic contains sulphur compounds which may lower blood cholesterol levels. These also have anti-cancer properties.

Haricot beans: similar to black-eye beans.

Kale is similar to broccoli, but generally contains even higher levels of the same micro-nutrients.

Kidney beans: similar to black-eye beans

Leeks: similar to onions

Lentils: similar to black-eye beans.

Mushrooms contain traces of chromium, which may be helpful in adult-onset diabetes.

Onions contain a flavonoid called quercitin, which has anti-inflammatory and cardio-protective properties. They also contain pre-biotic fibres, other dietary fibre, and some of the same sulphur compounds that are found in garlic. Red onions may contain slightly more quercitin than white.

Peppers (red, orange and yellow) contain flavonoids which are anti-inflammatory, and have cardio-protective and anti-cancer properties. The red peppers are, in addition, a good source of beta carotene.

The health benefits of selected foods

Potatoes have traces of Vitamin C and the B vitamins. They have a high glycemic index.

Shiitake mushrooms contain polysaccharide molecules which act as adjuvants, or immuno-stimulants. Similar compounds occur in Echinacea, pear skin and the cell walls of certain bacteria.

Spinach is a good source of beta carotene and Vitamin C, which may help to prevent cancers; lutein, which protects the eyes; Vitamin K, essential for maintaining healthy bones; dietary fibre; and betaine, a valuable compound that is both cardio-protective and immuno-supportive.

Sweet potatoes are a rich source of beta carotene; the deeper the colour, the higher the beta carotene content.

Wasabi (Japanese horseradish) contains traces of B vitamins and trace minerals.

Miscellaneous

Chocolate is now gaining acceptance as a health food, especially dark chocolate. This is due to its high content of anti-oxidant flavonoids, which are cardio-protective, cancer-protective and anti-inflammatory. The fat in chocolate (stearic acid) is metabolised in the body to oleic acid (as in olive oil), so that too may be cardio-protective. Chocolate contains a lot of calories, however, and the white and milk chocolates in particular have a high glycemic index (ie they increase blood sugar levels); so don't overdo.

Grape juice (especially red grape juice) is a good source of flavonoids shown to reduce platelet stickiness. Similar to red wine, but not quite as potent.

Green tea is another source of flavonoids, considered to be cardio-protective and cancer-protective. The combination of flavonoids and fluorides in tea probably help to ward off tooth and gum disease.

Groundnut oil: groundnuts are peanuts. Peanut oil is a reasonable source of MUFAs, which are cardio-protective.

Nori seaweed is a good source of minerals including iodine, zinc and copper. It also provides traces of calcium, iron, magnesium and potassium.

Olive oil contains mono-unsaturated fatty acids (MUFAs), which can help lower 'bad' cholesterol in the blood, and flavonoids which are reported to reduce the risk of colon and other cancers.

Salt: high sodium is a major cause of raised blood pressure. Switch from table salt to a low sodium/higher potassium and magnesium salt alternative to help reduce blood pressure.

Sesame oil/seeds contain MUFAs, Omega 6 PUFAs, Vitamin E and flavonoids.

Soy protein is derived from **soya beans** and has been proven to lower blood cholesterol levels. It must, therefore, be considered to be cardio-protective. Some soy extracts contain isoflavones reported to alleviate pre-menstrual and post-menopausal symptoms, which confer additional cardio- and some cancer protection. Some isoflavones (eg genistein) have additional anti-cancer properties. Last but not least, soy protein is of a very high quality; its amino acid composition means that it is regarded as a complete protein, similar to meat or egg, so is particularly suitable for vegetarians.

Sunflower oil is a source of Omega 6 PUFAs and some Vitamin E.

Wine: red wine contains flavonoids, anti-oxidant compounds with anti-inflammatory properties which reduce the risk of heart disease and cancers. White wine is not as good a source. For maximal flavonoid levels, choose a wine with the deepest red colouring: Cabernet Sauvignon grapes tend to score particularly highly.

Explanatory Notes

Anti-oxidant: A substance capable of neutralising free radicals, which could otherwise cause tissue damage in the body.

Carotenoids: A group of compounds derived from foods which have anti-oxidant, immuno-stimulating, anti-cancer and other health-promoting properties. Typically coloured, varying from red (lycopene, astaxanthin) to yellow (lutein) and orange (alpha and beta carotene).

Flavonoids: A group of compounds derived from foods which have anti-oxidant, anti-inflammatory, anti-bacterial and anti-vi properties. They are also anti-glycosyl nt, which means they help to reduce the cross nking of collagen and elastin which wou herwise lead to loss of elasticity of the sl arteries, etc.

Flavonoids are vital ingredients in our diet. Often coloured, they range from curcumin (yellow) to anthocyanins (typically red, blue and purple).

Glycemic index: The extent to which the carbohydrate elements in food increase blood sugar levels. Refined carbohydrates have a high glycemic index, while unrefined carbohydrates have, in general, a low one.

The high glycemic index of the Western diet has now been identified as a probable cause of Type 2 diabetes – so a shift to a lower GI diet is strongly recommended.

MUFAs: Mono-unsaturated fatty acids contain a single double bond and are liquid at room temperatures (eg olive, peanut oils). They help to lower LDL (the 'bad' cholesterol).

PUFAs: Poly-unsaturated fatty acids contain more than one double bond and are liquid at room temperature (eg sunflower, safflower oils).

Pre-biotic: A dietary fibre which stimulates the growth of bifidobacteria and other healthy bacteria in the gut.

Pro-biotic: Healthy bacteria, which are consumed either in fermented milk products or as supplements.

Quercitin: a flavonoid found in onions and apples. Probably the quantitatively most important flavonoid in the Western diet.

Saturated fats contain no double bonds. Solid at room temperature, they are mostly derived from meat and dairy foods. The only plant sources of saturated fats are coconuts and palm oil.

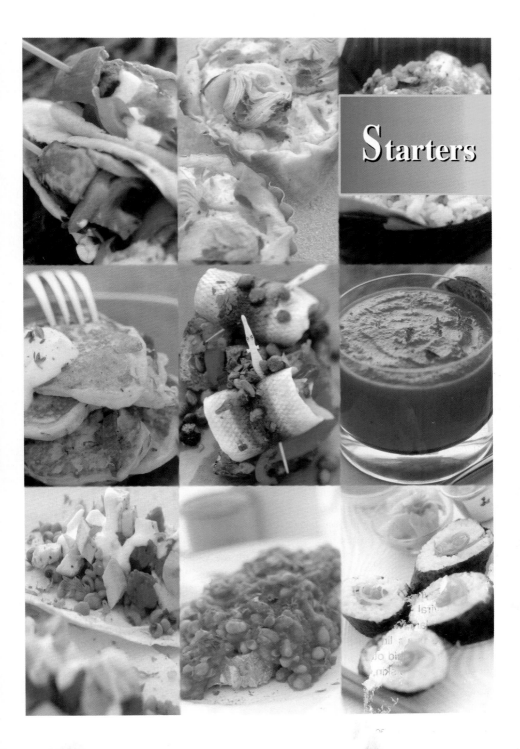

Starters

Baby spinach salad

**Serves 6 as a starter
or 4 as a light lunch**

Time Guide
Preparation: 10 mins
Cooking time: 25 mins

*450g/1lb baby spinach,
washed and spun dry*

*Unsmoked back bacon
1 rasher per person*

*2 medium red onions,
each cut into 6 wedges*

*30g/1oz Brazil nuts,
very roughly chopped*

4 free range eggs

*2 slices granary bread,
cut into croutons*

100ml extra virgin olive oil

40ml balsamic vinegar

Freshly ground black pepper

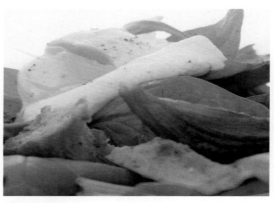

Method

1   Make the croutons. Toss the small cubes of bread in a little extra virgin olive oil and bake in the oven at GM6/200C for 5-7 minutes. (Keep your eye on them as they can suddenly burn!)

2   Turn the oven down to GM5/180C and roast the onion wedges for about 20 minutes.

3   In the meantime, grill the bacon until crispy and cut into strips.

4   In a large bowl combine the baby spinach, strips of crispy bacon and Brazil nuts.

5   On each plate, pile up some of the salad mixture and place a couple of pieces of the roasted onion on top. Drizzle with olive oil, balsamic vinegar and freshly ground black pepper.

6   Poach the eggs in a pan of simmering water and when ready place on top of the salad pile.

7   Sprinkle with the croutons.

DR CLAYTON SAYS:

Spinach is an excellent source of beta-carotene and Vitamin C, while **red onions** are rich in the flavonoid quercitin, thought to be one of the most powerful cardio-protective substances yet discovered.

...nuts are one of the best dietary sources of selenium. They also contain Omega 6 PUFAs, as well as the anti-oxidant Vitamin E, which are all cardio-protective.

Rollmop and caper-topped bruschetta

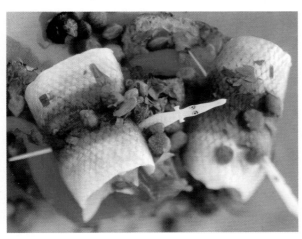

Serves 2 as a light lunch

Time Guide
Preparation: 5 mins
Cooking time: 45 mins

2 large slices of walnut bread (see baked bean and walnut bread recipe pp22-23)

Extra virgin olive oil

2 red peppers, cut in half, stalk and seeds removed

2 rollmops

2 tbsp capers

2 medium red onions, peeled and thinly sliced

Freshly ground black pepper

1 tsp freshly chopped parsley

Method

1 Place a little extra virgin olive oil in a small pan, add the thinly sliced red onions and place over a low heat until soft but not brown. They will caramelise and taste quite sweet.

2 In the meantime in a hot oven GM6/200C roast the red peppers in a little olive oil for 20-30 mins until the skins look quite charred. Remove and place in a bowl, tightly cover with cling film and allow to cool until the skins slide off fairly easily.

3 Drizzle the walnut bread with extra virgin olive oil and place in an oven GM6/200C or under a medium/hot grill until crisp and golden.

4 Top each slice of toasted bread with the red pepper cut into slithers, the red onion mixture and the rollmop, sprinkle over the capers, parsley and freshly ground black pepper.

5 Serve immediately, before the toast becomes soggy, with a spinach salad on the side.

DR CLAYTON SAYS:

Herrings are oily fish, an excellent source of Omega 3 for powerful protection against heart disease and osteoporosis (it helps the absorption of ca.

Red onions and red peppers both contain flavonoids which also protect against heart disease.

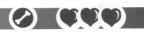

Lentil and spinach dhal

Serves 4

Time Guide
Preparation: 15 mins
Cooking time: 40 mins

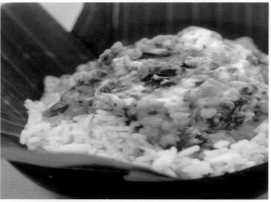

225g/8oz split lentils

400g/14oz fresh spinach,
washed well and drained

1 large onion, finely chopped

1 tbsp sunflower oil

2.5cm/1 inch piece root ginger,
peeled and grated

1 large clove of garlic, crushed

1 tbsp ground cumin

1 tbsp ground coriander

1 tsp ground turmeric

3-4 tbsp low fat live natural yoghurt

Low sodium salt and black pepper

225ml/1/2 pint vegetable stock

Method

1   Steam the spinach, drain well and chop.

2   Rinse the lentils in cold water and cover with fresh cold water in a pan and bring to the boil. Boil rapidly for 10 minutes.

3   Heat the sunflower oil in a pan and add the chopped onion and ginger, soften for 5 mins, then add the garlic and spices. Stir for at least 1 minute.

4   Add the cooked and drained lentils to the pan, cover with vegetable stock and cook for a further 15-20 minutes until tender. Add a little more stock or water if it looks dry.

5   Add the chopped spinach to the pan and heat through.

6   Finally add the yoghurt and season with low sodium salt and pepper.

7   Serve with Basmati rice and top with fresh coriander.

DR CLAYTON SAYS:

Some excellent anti-inflammatory ingredients are in this starter. **Spinach** contributes beta-carotene, lutein and Vitamin C, while **garlic** and **onions** contain sulphur compounds, all cancer-protective.

Both **ginger** flavonoids and **turmeric** (curcuminoids) have marked anti-inflammatory properties.

Lentils are a very good source of fibre, B vitamins, and carbohydrates with a low glycemic index.

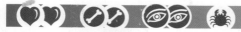

Curly kale gnocchi

Serves 4

Time Guide

Preparation:15 mins
Chilling time: 1 hour
Cooking time: 10 mins

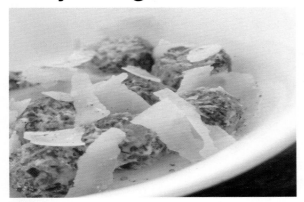

200g/7oz fresh kale, cooked, drained well and very finely chopped

1 large free range egg

200g/7oz ricotta or quark cheese

55g/2oz feta cheese, crumbled

Low sodium salt and black pepper

30g/1oz parmesan cheese, freshly grated

Extra virgin olive oil

Plain flour

Method

1   Mix together the quark or ricotta with the crumbled feta in a bowl with a fork. Mix in the cooked, chopped kale and the beaten egg. (Add a little plain flour if the mixture is too sloppy.) Taste for seasoning and if necessary add a little low sodium salt and black pepper.

2   With your hands shape this mixture into strawberry-sized shapes and roll them in seasoned flour. Put them in the fridge to firm up for about an hour.

3   Bring a pan of water to the boil and turn down to a simmer. Drop in a few gnocchi at a time; when they are ready they will bob to the surface.

4   Remove from the water with a slotted spoon and drain well. Arrange in a heat-proof dish, drizzle with extra virgin olive oil and sprinkle with parmesan.

5   Grill for 3-4 minutes until the cheese is turning golden and serve.

DR CLAYTON SAYS:

Kale, not unlike cabbage in its flavour and texture, is full of nutrition! It is an excellent source of Vitamin K, essential for healthy bones; sulphur compounds linked to cancer protection; the anti-oxidant Vitamin C; the flavonoid lutein, which protects the eyes; and dietary fibre.

Cheeses tend to be high in saturated fat, and often in salt too. Using the lower-fat types such as ricotta, feta and particularly quark, gets the benefit of their calcium and magnesium with less fat.

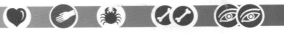

Chicken tortilla wraps

**Serves 8 as a starter
or 4 as a light lunch**

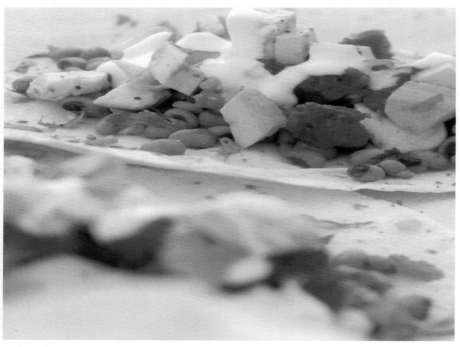

Filling

2 ripe avocados

Juice of half a lemon

1 x 200g/7oz tub low fat crème fraiche

1 bunch fresh coriander, three-quarters chopped roughly, one quarter reserved for garnish

2 chicken breasts, skin and all fat removed, cut into finger-sized strips

1x 400g/14oz tin black-eye beans, drained and rinsed

Low sodium salt

Freshly ground black pepper

Salsa style sauce

1 x 400g/14oz tin of tomatoes

1 tbsp tomato puree

1 small onion

2 cloves garlic, chopped

2 red chillies, de-seeded and chopped

Pinch of cayenne pepper

1 tsp golden caster sugar

Low sodium salt and black pepper to taste

1 pack tortilla wraps (8)

Method

Time Guide
Preparation: 15 mins
Cooking time: 30 mins

1   Start by making the salsa style sauce. Sweat onions and garlic in a little extra virgin olive oil until soft but not brown. Next add the tomato puree, cayenne pepper, sugar and chopped chillies, then add the tinned tomatoes and cook until a thick pulpy consistency. Season with low sodium salt as necessary.

2   In a non-stick frying pan drizzle a few drops of extra virgin olive oil, add the chicken strips and fry for about 3-4 minutes until cooked, add the beans and stir to heat through. Finally add the chopped coriander.

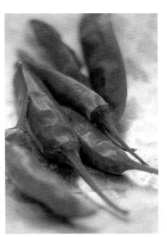

3   Slice the avocado lengthways and drizzle with lemon juice to avoid discolouration.

4   Assemble the tortillas: lay each tortilla on a plate and place some of the chicken mixture along the centre, top with a little of the tomato salsa, a slice of avocado and finish with a teaspoon of crème fraiche. Then roll up. Continue with all the tortillas.

5   Place one or two on each plate and top with sprigs of fresh coriander.

DR CLAYTON SAYS:

A great synergistic combination of key micro-nutrients. **Avocados** are rich in Vitamin E, a key anti-oxidant against heart disease and free radical damage. They also contain potassium, which can help to lower blood pressure.

Tomatoes are a rich source of Vitamin C, as well as lycopene, a powerful carotenoid which enhances the immune system and fights cancer cells; and chromium which may help against diabetes.

Black-eye beans are full of fibre, as well as B vitamins, and are a good source of low-glycemic-index carbohydrates.

Garlic, onions, coriander and **chillies** all contain protective ingredients (see food list). Use them all liberally in your cooking.

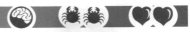

Mediterranean pancakes

**Serves 4
(makes 8 pancakes)**

Time Guide
Preparation: 25 mins
Cooking time: 10-12 mins

450g/1lb tub low fat fromage frais

125g/4¹/₂oz self-raising flour

2 free range eggs

1 tbsp fresh chopped thyme or oregano

1 tbsp fresh chopped parsley

55g/2oz freshly grated parmesan cheese

6 sundried tomatoes, cut into slivers

Extra virgin olive oil

Freshly ground black pepper

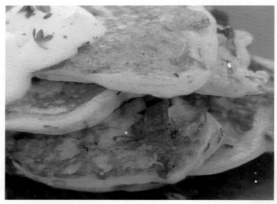

Method

1   Sift the flour into a large bowl, make a well in the centre and break the eggs into it. With a balloon whisk mix together and then add the fromage frais. Mix well to form a stiff batter. If very stiff, add a tablespoon of skimmed milk. Season this batter well with black pepper.

2   Next stir in the parmesan, sundried tomatoes and herbs. Taste for seasoning, adding a little low sodium salt if necessary, and leave to stand for about 10-15 minutes.

3   Heat a little olive oil in a non-stick frying pan. Make each pancake with a couple of tablespoons of the mixture, flattening slightly with the back of a spoon. Cook two or three at a time over a medium heat for a few minutes on each side, until brown. When cooked put in a warming oven, until you have finished the whole batch.

4   Serve immediately with a side salad and/or some lean, crispy, grilled bacon.

DR CLAYTON SAYS:

Eggs contain lecithin phospholipids which increase levels of HDL cholesterol (the 'good' cholesterol) and anti-cancer carotenoids. The more intensely coloured the yolk, the higher the carotenoid content; free range eggs generally contain higher levels.

Tomatoes contain lycopene, a flavonoid with strong anti-cancer and cardio-protective properties.

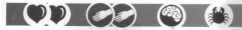

Bacon, artichoke and quark tarts

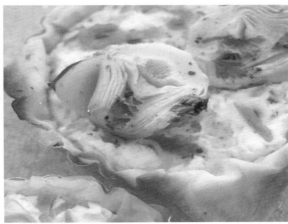

Serves 4 as a light lunch

Time Guide
Preparation: 10-15 mins
Cooking time: 25 mins

4 sheets filo pastry

Extra virgin olive oil

3 rashers lean unsmoked back bacon, cut into thin strips

1 tbsp fresh thyme, chopped

1 small leek, chopped finely

4 artichoke hearts, cut in half

1 x 250g/9oz tub quark, virtually fat free soft cheese

Low sodium salt and freshly ground black pepper

Method

1   Fry the strips of bacon in a drizzle of olive oil, then add the leeks and allow to sweat until soft. Remove from the heat.

2   On a board, lightly brush a sheet of filo pastry with a little olive oil. Cut into squares large enough to line four individual tartlet tins. Continue to do this until the cases have four layers of filo in them. The last sheet should NOT be oiled.

3   In a bowl, mash the quark with a fork and mix in the chopped thyme, leeks and bacon. Season with a little low sodium salt and black pepper to taste.

4   Divide the cheesy mixture between the four tartlet cases and top each one with two halves of artichoke heart.

5   Bake in a preheated oven GM5/190C for about 15 minutes, until the pastry is crisp and golden. Serve immediately with a small salad.

DR CLAYTON SAYS:

Leeks contain quercitin, which has anti-inflammatory and cardio-protective properties, as well as pre-biotic and other types of dietary fibre, which protect the lower bowel.

Quark is a good low-fat source of calcium.

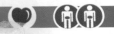

Wild salmon sushi

Serves 4

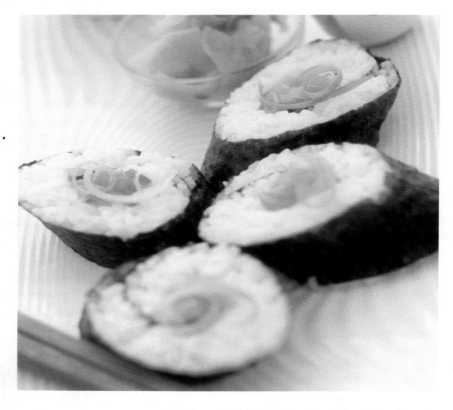

Time Guide

Preparation: 15-20 mins
Cooking time: 20 mins
plus cooling

1 skinned fillet of wild salmon (very fresh), cut into long, thin strips

1 packet Nori seaweed sheets

2¹/₂ cups sushi rice

Rice wine vinegar to taste

Half a cucumber, core removed, cut lengthways into thin strips

Bunch of spring onions, trimmed and cut into long thin strips

To serve: soy sauce, pickled ginger, wasabi (Japanese horseradish)

Method

1   Cook the sushi rice according to the instructions on the packet. While still hot dress with rice wine vinegar to season.

2   On a sushi mat (a small rolling mat available from Asian foodshops or cookshops) lay a sheet of Nori seaweed, cover with a layer of the cooled sushi rice, leaving a 1cm($1/2$ inch) border around the edge.

3   With the handle of a wooden spoon make an indentation in the rice. Into this lay a strip of cucumber and a strip of spring onion, and top with salmon.

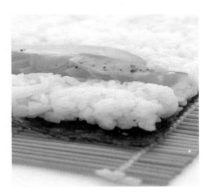

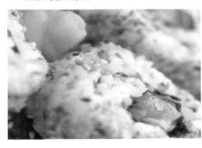

4   Moisten the edge with a little cold water and roll up the sushi tightly like a swiss roll.

5   Trim each roll and cut into 4cm ($1^1/_2$ inch) lengths. This may be done on the diagonal and the rolls stood up on their ends.

6   Serve with small dishes of pickled ginger, soy sauce and wasabi.

DR CLAYTON SAYS:

Wild salmon is an excellent source of Omega 3 fatty acids to protect the heart from coronary artery disease, as well as help absorption of calcium to help prevent osteoporosis. Wild salmon is also rich in iodine and astaxanthin, a carotenoid derived from red algae, whence its colour.

Salmon also contains Vitamin D, which is essential for the body to take up calcium and distribute it in the body.

Nori seaweed is a good source of essential minerals, including iodine, zinc, copper, iron, magnesium and potassium. Iodine is essential for the normal functioning of the thyroid gland. In the many people who are depleted in copper and iron, these minerals have a variety of health-giving properties, including anti-oxidant and blood-building effects.

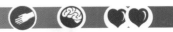

'Simply red' soup

Serves 4

Time Guide
Preparation: 15 mins
Cooking time: 60 mins

10 plum tomatoes, halved

2 uncooked beetroot, peeled and quartered

2 large red onions, peeled and quartered

3 red peppers, halved and seeds removed

2 carrots, peeled and cut into chunks

2 large cloves garlic, whole, unpeeled

2 tbsp tomato puree

1 litre/2 pints vegetable stock

50g/2oz red split lentils

Chopped herbs, such as marjoram, parsley or oregano

Low sodium salt and black pepper

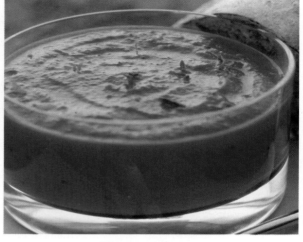

DR CLAYTON SAYS:

This soup is packed full of carotenoids (which give yellow, red and orange colours to fruit and vegetables), particularly beta-carotene and lycopene, and the anti-oxidant Vitamin C.

Red split lentils are a good source of fibre and protein, and also lower blood cholesterol levels. **Herbs** such as **thyme** are also anti-oxidants. All in all, a powerful combination of micro-nutrients against the main degenerative diseases.

Method

1   In a medium oven (GM5/190C) roast the first 6 ingredients in roasting tins drizzled with olive oil for about 30 minutes.

2   Remove from the oven and transfer to a large saucepan. Add the vegetable stock and rinsed red lentils, and cook for a further 20-30 minutes until the lentils are soft. Stir in the tomato puree and liquidize, adding more water or stock if necessary.

3   Season the soup to taste with low sodium salt and black pepper.

4   Ladle into warm bowls and top with chopped herbs. Serve with warm granary bread.

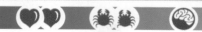

Broccoli terrine

Makes 1 loaf tin

Method

1 Line a large loaf tin with non-stick baking parchment.

2 Sweat the onion and garlic until soft in a little olive oil, do not allow to brown.

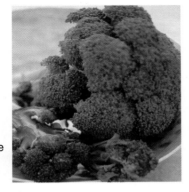

3 In a food processor, puree the broccoli, onions, garlic, parsley, egg yolks and cottage cheese together.

4 Transfer to a bowl and stir in the breadcrumbs, pesto and parmesan and season as necessary with black pepper and low sodium salt.

5 Beat the egg white until stiff, loosen the broccoli mixture with a spoonful of the egg whites and then fold in the rest carefully.

6 Turn into the lined loaf tin and bake at GM6/200C for about 25-30 mins until set.

7 Allow to cool before cutting into slices.

Time Guide

Preparation: 20 mins
Cooking time: 40 mins

450g/1lb fresh broccoli, steamed and drained

1 large onion, chopped

1 clove garlic, chopped

2 free range eggs, separated

1 tbsp fresh chopped parsley

250g/9oz very low fat cottage cheese

2 large or 3 small slices wholemeal bread, made into breadcrumbs

5 tbsp freshly grated parmesan cheese

1 tbsp pesto (preferably fresh home made)

A pinch of low sodium salt

Freshly ground black pepper

DR CLAYTON SAYS:

Broccoli is an excellent source of several protective nutrients: Vitamin K, for healthy bones, sulphur compounds linked to cancer protection, the anti-oxidant Vitamin C, lutein which protects the eyes, and dietary fibre.

Onions, garlic and **herbs** all contribute to protection against heart disease and cancer.

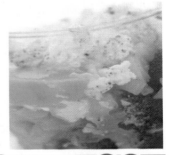

  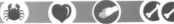

Homemade baked beans on walnut bread

Serves 4 as a light lunch

Time Guide
Preparation: 45 mins
Cooking time: 2 hours
15 mins to allow rising
time for bread

225g/8oz dried haricot beans

Tomato sauce
1 x 500ml carton of passata (sieved tomatoes)

1 tbsp tomato puree

1 medium onion, chopped

1 large clove garlic, crushed

1 tbsp extra virgin olive oil

1 tbsp chopped fresh thyme

1 tbsp chopped fresh oregano

1 tsp chopped fresh parsley

1 tsp golden caster sugar

A little vegetable stock

Low sodium salt

Freshly ground black pepper

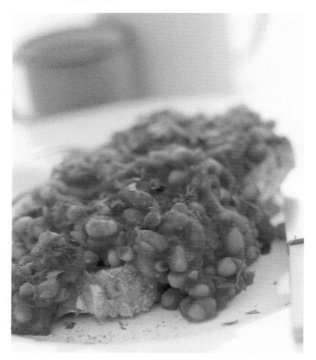

Method for the 'baked' beans

1   Soak the haricot beans overnight, boil for 10 minutes and simmer until tender.

2   Sweat the onions in the extra virgin olive oil until soft and transparent. Add the crushed garlic and cook for 1 minute. Add the tomato puree, the passata and the boiled haricot beans, plus sugar and a little vegetable stock to thin the sauce slightly.

3   Cook the above for about 30 minutes, stir in the fresh herbs and season with low sodium salt and black pepper.

4   Toast sliced bread, top with beans and serve immediately.

Method for the walnut bread

1 First dissolve the yeast in about half of the warm water.

2 Mix the granary and white flours in a large bowl and make a well in the centre. Pour in the dissolved yeast, the remaining warm water and the extra virgin olive oil. Mix together with a knife or wooden spoon. When all ingredients are incorporated knead the dough until soft and elastic, flouring the board lightly if necessary.

3 Put this dough in a lightly floured bowl and leave to rise in a warm place for about 1 hour, until doubled in size.

4 Knock back (knead again to get rid of any large pockets of air in the dough), add the walnuts at this stage and knead in to distribute evenly through the dough. Shape into a round and place on a baking sheet to rise again until about $1^1/_2$ times original size.

5 When ready, bake at GM6/200C for about 40 minutes. Check to see if the loaf is cooked by tapping the base (when it is ready it will sound hollow). Allow to cool on a rack.

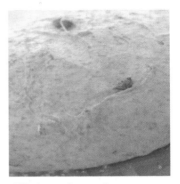

Walnut bread

30g/1oz fresh yeast

225ml /$^1/_2$ pint warm water

225g/8oz strong white flour

225g/8oz granary flour preferably with added wheatgerm

1 tsp low sodium salt

$2^1/_2$ tbsp extra virgin olive oil

55g/2oz walnuts, roughly chopped

Freshly ground black pepper

DR CLAYTON SAYS:

Haricot beans are a good low-fat source of protein and also provide minerals and B vitamins. They help to control blood sugar levels and can be useful to diabetics and may also help to lower cholesterol levels.

Tomatoes in any form are rich in Vitamin C, and lycopene, a powerful anti-cancer carotenoid.

The granary flour in the walnut bread is an excellent source of insoluble dietary fibre. And the walnuts have a high Vitamin E content, which may be cardio-protective.

Marinated chicken kebabs

Serves 2

Chicken

2 chicken breasts, skin removed and fat trimmed away, cut into cubes and marinated for at least 4 hours in the following marinade:

> *Juice of half a lemon*
>
> *2 tsp turmeric*
>
> *2 cloves garlic, crushed*
>
> *Freshly ground black pepper*
>
> *Extra virgin olive oil*
>
> *2 tsp cumin*
>
> *2 tsp ground coriander*

For the kebabs

1 small red pepper, deseeded and cut into squares

1 small yellow pepper, deseeded and cut into squares

1 small green pepper, deseeded and cut into squares

6 button mushrooms, cleaned

2 pitta bread

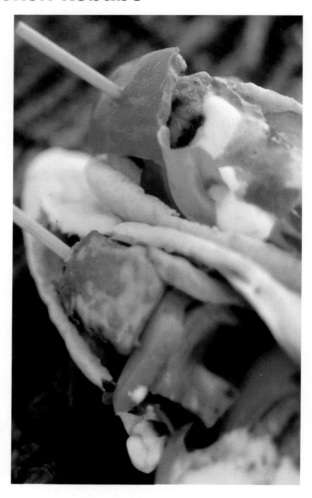

Cucumber and yoghurt dip

7.5cm/3 inch length of cucumber, finely diced

150ml/¹/₄ pint carton live natural low fat yoghurt

1 tbsp fresh chopped mint

Low sodium salt and black pepper

Method

1 Mix together all the marinade ingredients and leave the cubed chicken to marinate in the fridge for at least 4 hours.

2 Thread onto skewers (or stripped rosemary stalks) alternating the mushrooms and peppers with the chicken.

3 Grill the kebabs under a medium/hot grill for 4-5 minutes each side. Check that the chicken is cooked through. Cook for longer if necessary, but avoid charring the meat as this creates carcinogens.

4 Serve with cucumber dip or mango chutney and grilled pitta bread.

5 Alternatively serve with steamed broccoli and Basmati rice.

Time Guide

Preparation: 15 mins

Marinating: 4 hours

Cooking time: 12 mins

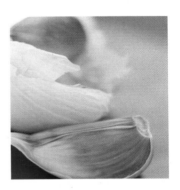

DR CLAYTON SAYS:

A delicious variant on the kebab theme, which shows that fast food can also be healthy food. Take care not to char the meat, however, as this produces carcinogens.

Peppers contain flavonoids which are anti-inflammatory, and have cardio-protective and anti-cancer properties.

Red peppers are also a good source of beta carotene.

Turmeric provides a group of flavonoids called curcuminoids, which have many therapeutic properties, including anti-inflammatory, cardio-protective, anti-diabetic and anti-cancer.

Jerusalem artichoke soup

Serves 4

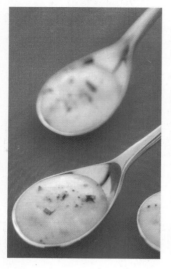

1 medium onion, chopped

2 tbsp extra virgin olive oil

1½ lb/675g Jerusalem artichokes

500ml/1 pint skimmed milk

500ml/1 pint vegetable stock

Low sodium salt

Freshly ground black pepper

4 tbsp live natural yoghurt

Chopped parsley

Time Guide

Preparation: 10 mins

Cooking time: 40 mins

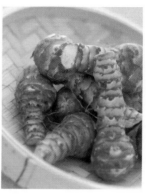

Method

1   Heat the olive oil in a large pan and sweat the onion until soft and transparent.

2   Peel the Jerusalem artichokes like potatoes and put in a bowl of acidulated water (water with a little vinegar or lemon juice) to prevent the artichokes discolouring.

3   Slice the artichokes and add to the pan. Sweat the artichokes with the onions for about 5 mins. Next add the hot vegetable stock and skimmed milk, season with black pepper and simmer gently for about 25 mins.

4   When artichokes are tender liquidise the soup and check the seasoning, season with low sodium salt and pepper to taste.

5   To serve: ladle into hot bowls, top with a teaspoon of live yoghurt and sprinkle with chopped parsley.

DR CLAYTON SAYS:

Jerusalem artichokes, despite their unpre-possessing appearance, are an unrivalled source of inulin, a pre-biotic which protects the lower bowel, liver and heart.

Live yoghurt contains pro-biotic bacteria. Not all of these are effective, but those in certain ranges of yoghurts seem to be able to protect against gastrointestinal infections.

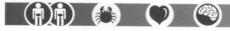

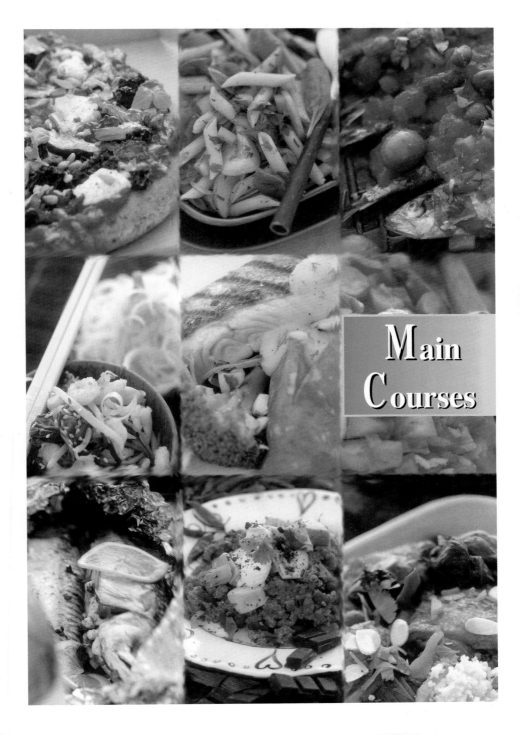

Main Courses

Chilli sans carne

Serves 4

Time Guide
Preparation: 10-15 mins
Cooking time: 50 mins

120g/4¹/₂oz dry weight
soya mince
(480g approx. when
reconstituted)

2 onions, chopped

2 cloves garlic, crushed

1 tsp chilli powder

2 tbsp tomato puree

1 x 400g/14oz tin
chopped tomatoes

Extra virgin olive oil

1 x 400g/14oz tin black-
eye beans or red kidney
beans, drained

Low sodium salt, to taste

30g/1oz very dark
chocolate (70% cocoa
solids)

Avocado salsa

1 avocado pear

1 tbsp fresh coriander,
chopped

Lemon juice

Extra virgin olive oil

4 tbsp low fat crème
fraiche

Brown rice to serve

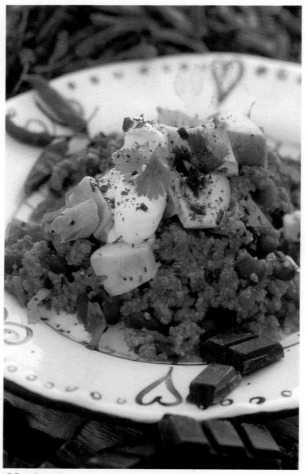

Method

1   Soak the dried soya mince in boiling water for
    about a minute, then drain well.

2   In a large frying pan heat a little extra virgin olive
    oil and fry the onions over a low/medium heat until
    lightly browned, then add the garlic.

3   To this add the drained mince and continue to fry for a few minutes.

4   Add the chilli powder and fry for another minute before adding the tomato puree and tinned tomatoes. Cover and allow to simmer for about 30 minutes. Add the drained tinned beans to the pan and continue to cook for a further 15 minutes or so uncovered.

5   In the meantime, peel and stone the avocado. Then cut into tiny dice, sprinkle with lemon juice to avoid discolouration and mix with the chopped coriander and a drizzle of olive oil.

6   Taste the chilli and season well with the grated chocolate and low sodium salt.

7   Serve on a bed of brown rice topped with a spoonful of crème fraiche and a little of the avocado salsa.

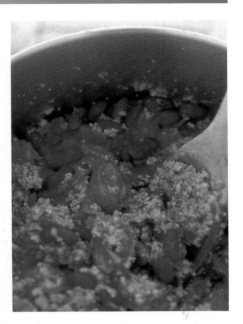

WHAT DR CLAYTON SAYS

The combination of ingredients in this recipe has both cancer-protective and cardio-protective properties.

Soy protein lowers cholesterol levels and contains important anti-cancer isoflavones.

More heart protection comes from the anti-oxidant flavonoids in dark chocolate, the mono- and poly-unsaturated fats in avocados, and of course tomatoes, which are the richest source of the carotenoid lycopene. Lycopene also has anti-cancer properties, as do the anti-oxidants in chillies.

Black-eye or kidney beans are a good source of fibre and B vitamins, and provide low glycemic index carbohydrates which can protect against adult-onset diabetes.

Real food pizza

Serves 4

Time Guide
Preparation: 45 mins
Cooking time: 1 hour

Pizza base

170g/6oz wholewheat flour

55g/2oz strong white flour

$1/2$ tsp low sodium salt

$1/2$ tbsp fresh thyme or oregano

Freshly ground black pepper

170ml/6floz warm water

1 tsp sugar

1 tsp dried yeast

Tomato sauce

Extra virgin olive oil

1 onion, chopped finely

1 clove garlic, crushed

1 tsp tomato puree

1 x 400g/14oz tin chopped plum tomatoes

Low sodium salt and black pepper

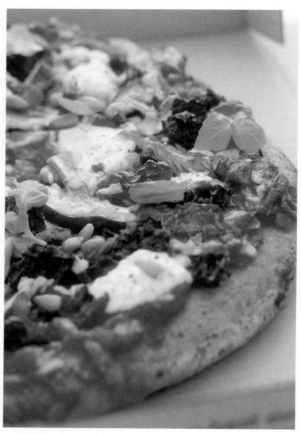

Topping

55g/2oz shiitake mushrooms, sliced

110g/4oz quark soft cheese

About 100g/4oz kale, washed, steamed and chopped finely

4 sundried tomatoes, sliced

30g/1oz pine nuts

30g/1oz parmesan cheese, freshly grated

Handful fresh basil

Method

To make the dough:

1 In a bowl mix together the yeast, warm water and sugar and leave in a warm place to froth.

2 In a separate bowl mix together the flours, herbs and seasonings.

3 When the yeast is frothy, mix with the flours. Knead for a few minutes to give a soft, non-sticky dough.

4 Roll out into a 22.5cm/9 inch round and place on a baking sheet and cover lightly with a clean tea towel. Leave for about 30 minutes.

To make the sauce:

1 Sweat the onion in a little olive oil and add the garlic. Add the tomato puree and tinned tomatoes.

2 Cook down to a pulp and season with low sodium salt and freshly ground black pepper.

To assemble:

1 On the bread base spread the tomato sauce. Scatter a layer of kale over the sauce and dollop spoonfuls of the quark cheese over the top. Sprinkle over the shiitake, pinenuts, sundried tomatoes and finally the parmesan.

2 Bake at the top of a hot oven at GM6/200C for about 20-25 minutes until the base is crisp.

3 Garnish with torn basil leaves and freshly ground black pepper. Serve immediately.

DR CLAYTON SAYS:

Definitely not a junk food, this pizza has lots of multi-function protective ingredients.

Tomatoes contain lycopene, cardio-protective and anti-cancer; onions have the flavonoid quercitin with anti-inflammatory and cardio-protective properties; kale is an excellent source of Vitamin K for bone health, as well as containing the anti-oxidant Vitamin C, sulphur compounds and lutein, which protects the eyes.

Shiitake mushrooms contain polysaccharide molecules which help to stimulate the immune system, and thyme is capable of activating the body's own detoxifying enzyme defences.

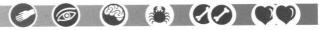

Mackerel kedgeree

Serves 4

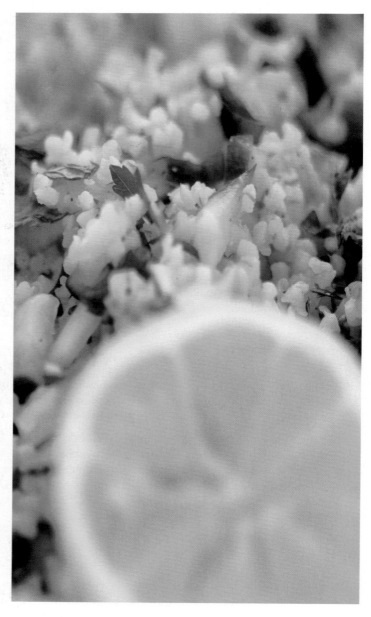

225g/8oz dry weight rice, cooked, well drained and cooled

2-3 smoked mackerel fillets (depending on size)

1 onion

1 tsp butter

Extra virgin olive oil

2 tbsp chopped parsley

$^1/_2$ tsp turmeric

$^1/_2$ tsp ground cumin

$^1/_2$ tsp ground coriander

$^1/_2$ tsp chilli powder

Lemon juice

2 large free range eggs, hard boiled, peeled and chopped

Low sodium salt and black pepper

Method

1   In a pan soften the onion in the butter and a little olive oil. Stir in the spices and cook for at least one minute.

2   Add the cooked rice and a little more olive oil if too dry.

3   Add the flaked fish, parsley, chopped eggs. Season with low sodium salt, pepper and a little lemon juice.

4   Warm through over a moderate heat, stirring to prevent sticking.

5   Serve immediately.

Time Guide

Preparation: 15 mins
or 1 hour to allow rice
to cook and cool

Cooking time: 5 mins

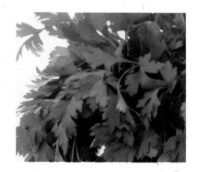

DR CLAYTON SAYS:

There are strongly cardio-protective ingredients in this recipe. **Mackerel** are an excellent source of Omega 3 PUFAs, which have strong cardio-protective properties. They have also been shown to reduce inflammation of the airways and joints, and can help to reduce the symptoms of asthma and arthritis. They also contain iodine (essential for thyroid function); traces of selenium; and a useful combination of calcium and Vitamin D, which can help to maintain healthy bones.

Eggs contain lecithin phospholipids which increase levels of HDL (the good cholesterol), and carotenoids. The more intensely coloured the yolk, the higher the carotenoid content; free range eggs generally contain higher levels of these valuable micro-nutrients. They have anti-cancer properties, and protect the eyes and skin.

Onions contain a flavonoid called quercitin, which has anti-inflammatory and cardio-protective properties. Onions also contain pre-biotic fibres, other dietary fibre, and some of the same sulphur compounds that are found in garlic.

Turmeric provides a group of flavonoids called curcuminoids, which have many therapeutic properties. They include anti-inflammatory, cardio-protective, anti-diabetic and anti-cancer activities.

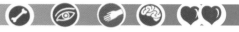

Scandinavian salmon

Serves 2

Time Guide
Preparation: 10 mins
Cooking time: 1 hour 10 mins

*2 pieces wild
salmon fillet*

2 sweet potatoes

*1 head broccoli cut
into florets*

*55g/2oz roughly
chopped Brazil nuts*

*Extra virgin olive
oil*

Black pepper

Dressing

*2-3 tbsp smooth
mustard*

1 tbsp sugar

*$1/2$ tsp low sodium
salt*

*1 tbsp white wine
vinegar*

*150ml/$^1/_4$ pint
sunflower oil*

*2-3 tbsp chopped
fresh dill*

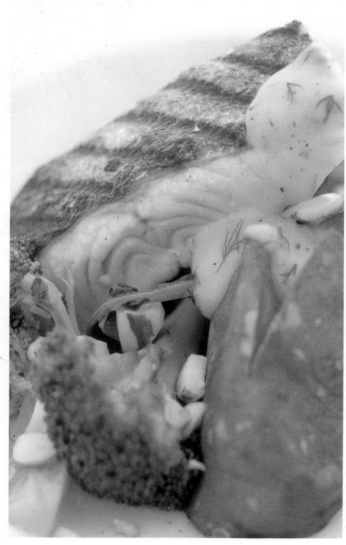

Method

1 Wash, prick and bake the sweet potatoes, as regular potatoes, in a hot oven for about 1 hour.

2 Heat a griddle pan or frying pan and add a little olive oil. When hot add the salmon skin side down to sear it and give it a nice colour.

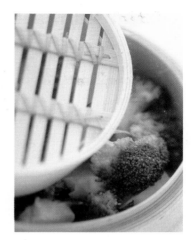

   Do not try and move it around; when it is ready it will lift out of the pan easily. Turn over and cook the other side.

   How long you cook it is up to you; some people like their salmon quite rare, others well cooked.

3 While doing this put the broccoli on to steam.

4 Make the dressing. Mix the mustard, sugar, low sodium salt and vinegar together, and then add the oil by degrees, slowly beating after each addition. Finally add the dill.

5 Serve the salmon with the sweet potato sprinkled with black pepper, broccoli sprinkled with olive oil, and Brazil nuts. Drizzle the sauce over the salmon.

DR CLAYTON SAYS:

Another healthy fish dish, particularly if it is wild salmon and the darkest red you can get. The combination of polyunsaturated fatty acids from the salmon, Brazil nuts and sunflower oil is strongly cardio-protective.

Salmon provide Omega 3 PUFAs, while **sunflower oil** provides Omega 6 PUFAs. This combination, together with the Vitamin E in **Brazil nuts**, is cardio-proective. The selenium in **Brazil nuts** confers additional cardio-protection and has anti-cancer properties.

Sweet potatoes provide dietary fibre, and traces of B vitamins, as well as beta carotene in the darker orange varieties.

Broccoli is an excellent source of Vitamin K, essential for healthy bones; sulphur compounds linked to cancer protection; the anti-oxidant Vitamin C; lutein, which protects the eyes, and dietary fibre.

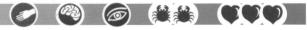

Vegetarian goulash

Serves 4

1 tbsp extra virgin olive oil

1 large onion, sliced

1 clove garlic, crushed

$\frac{1}{2}$ tbsp plain flour

1 tbsp paprika

$\frac{1}{4}$ tsp cayenne pepper

1x 400g/14oz tin chopped tomatoes

1 tbsp tomato puree

170g/6oz carrots, peeled and cut into chunks

170g/6oz new potatoes, cut into chunks

1 small red pepper de-seeded and chopped

1 small yellow pepper de-seeded and chopped

170g/6oz broccoli florets

225g/8oz courgettes, cut into chunks

55g/2oz shiitake mushrooms sliced

6-8 tbsp low fat crème fraiche

Low sodium salt and black pepper

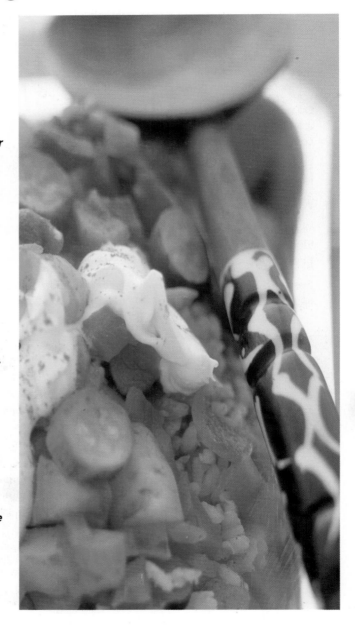

Method

1   Heat the oil in a large pan and fry the onion. Then add the crushed garlic, stir in the flour, paprika and cayenne, and continue stirring for a couple of minutes.

2   Stir in the tomato puree and tinned tomatoes.

3   Bring this mixture up to boiling point, add the prepared carrots, potatoes and red and yellow peppers and season with low sodium salt and pepper. Cover and continue to cook for about 20 minutes.

4   Add the remaining vegetables and cook for a further 10-15 minutes until the vegetables are 'al dente'. (Add a little more water if the mixture looks as though it is drying out.)

5   At the end of the cooking time, stir in the crème fraiche and sprinkle with a little more paprika.

6   Serve with brown rice.

Time Guide

Preparation: 15 mins
Cooking time: 50 mins

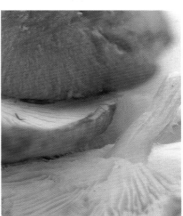

DR CLAYTON SAYS:

The vegetables in this dish contribute flavonoids, carotenoids, Vitamin C and dietary fibre, which have protective properties against the major degenerative diseases.

Tomatoes and **tomato products** are the richest source of lycopene, a carotenoid with strong cardio-protective and anti-cancer properties.

Carrots contain, as the name implies, beta carotene. Darker red carrots contain higher levels of this micro-nutrient.

Broccoli is an excellent source of Vitamin K, essential for healthy bones; sulphur compounds linked to cancer protection; the anti-oxidant Vitamin C; lutein, which protects the eyes, and dietary fibre.

Peppers (red, orange and yellow) contain flavonoids which are anti-inflammatory, and have cardio-protective and anti-cancer properties.

Shiitake mushrooms contain polysaccharides which act as immuno-stimulants.

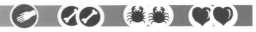

Oriental soya bean rice

Serves 4

Time Guide

Preparation: 20 mins

or 1 hour to allow rice to cook and cool

Cooking time: 20 mins

Sesame oil

110g/4oz bean-sprouts

225g/8oz dry weight brown rice – cooked and cooled

2 carrots, peeled and grated

4 spring onions, trimmed and chopped

1 large clove garlic, crushed

1.5cm/$^1/_2$ inch piece root ginger, peeled and grated

1 x 400g/14oz can soya beans, rinsed and drained

1 head broccoli, broken into florets and lightly steamed

2 free range eggs, lightly beaten

1 tbsp sesame seeds

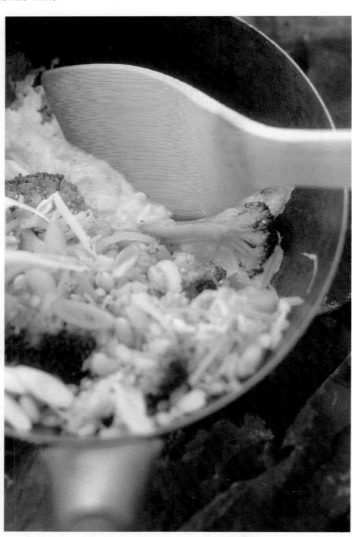

Method

1 Heat a wok and add a little sesame oil.

2 Stir fry the rice, carrots, garlic, three quarters of the spring onions, ginger, soya beans and beansprouts.

3 When heated through thoroughly, add the broccoli and eggs and continue to stir for another minute or so until the egg has set in thin strands.

4 Sprinkle with soy sauce to season.

5 Spoon into warm bowls and sprinkle over sesame seeds and remaining spring onions.

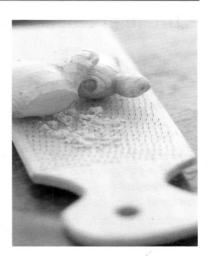

DR CLAYTON SAYS:

This recipe represents all that's best in nutrition, with a particular emphasis on protection against cancer.

Soya beans contain genistein, an isoflavone which not only inhibits cancer cells, it can also force them to revert to normal. Isoflavones offer protection against many types of cancers by inhibiting the growth of new blood vessels, which starve the cancers before they get the chance to grow.

Brown rice is an excellent source of dietary fibre essential for the healthy functioning of the gut.

Spring onions are a source of the anti-cancer flavonoid quercitin and also aid digestion and a healthy gut.

Broccoli is a rich source of Vitamin K, essential for bone repair and continual replacement of the skeleton. It is also an excellent source of Vitamin C, beta-carotene, folate, iron and potassium (which helps to lower blood pressure). It helps to speed up the body's own production of protective anti-oxidant enzymes and has anti-cancer properties.

Sesame seeds are a source of Vitamin E and calcium. **Ginger** is a powerful anti-oxidant and anti-inflammatory, which can be useful to sufferers of arthritis.

Carrots are a good source of beta-carotene essential for healthy vision. **Garlic** lowers 'bad' LDL cholesterol and is a powerful anti-oxidant.

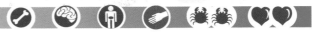

Moroccan chicken tagine served with couscous

Serves 4

Time Guide
Preparation: 20 mins
Marinating time: 4 hours
Cooking time: 35-40 mins

Tagine

8 chicken thighs, skin removed and fat trimmed

Marinated for up to 4 hours in:

> *6 tbsp extra virgin olive oil*
>
> *2 tsp turmeric*
>
> *1 tbsp ground cinnamon*
>
> *Juice and zest of 1 orange*
>
> *1 onion chopped*
>
> *2 tbsp chopped, fresh coriander*
>
> *2 cloves garlic, crushed*

2 onions, cut into quarters (trim off the hairy root, but leave the core in so that wedges do not fall apart)

2 tsp ground coriander

1 glass red wine

24 stoned prunes

A few fresh coriander leaves to garnish

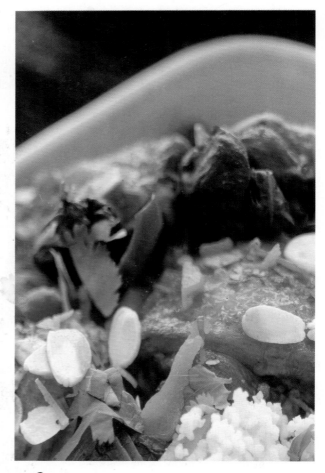

Couscous

300g/10oz couscous

16 dried apricots

30g/1oz flaked almonds, lightly toasted

Freshly ground black pepper

Low sodium salt

2 tbsp very roughly chopped fresh coriander

Method

1 While the chicken is marinating, prepare the other ingredients.

2 In a heavy bottomed casserole (hob and oven proof) heat a couple of tablespoons of olive oil in the pan and fry off the chicken thighs until lightly golden.

3 Add the wedges of onion, and continue to cook for a further 3-4 minutes turning as necessary to prevent the onions browning. Add the marinade ingredients to the pan, fry the ground coriander for a minute or two. Then add about 100ml water and the glass of red wine.

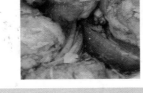

4 Cover with a well-fitting lid and cook for a further 20 minutes, over a low/medium heat to allow the chicken to cook through. Add the prunes to the pan, adding a little more water if necessary. Cover again and cook for a further 5-10 minutes.

5 Steam or soak the couscous according to the instructions on the packet. Stir through the dried apricots, chopped coriander and flaked almonds. Season to taste with a little low sodium salt and black pepper.

6 Serve the tagine on a bed of couscous and top with fresh coriander. Serve with green beans or spinach.

DR CLAYTON SAYS:

The Moroccans have one of the lowest rates of death from heart disease in the world! This is a variation on the traditional Moroccan 'tagine'.

The fruits contain a range of flavonoids. **Citrus fruit** (oranges, lemons, grapefruit) flavonoids are anti-inflammatory, cardio-protective, and probably anti-cancer. **Prunes** also give high levels of flavonoids, and **apricots** contain carotenoids, specifically beta carotene.

Red wine also contains flavonoids with cardio-protective and anti-cancer properties.

The flavonoid quercitin, found in **onions**, has anti-inflammatory and cardio-protective properties. They also contain pre-biotic fibres, other dietary fibre, and some of the same sulphur compounds that are found in garlic.

Roasted vegetables with cracked wheat salad

Time Guide

Serves 4

Preparation: 30 mins

Cooking time: 30 mins

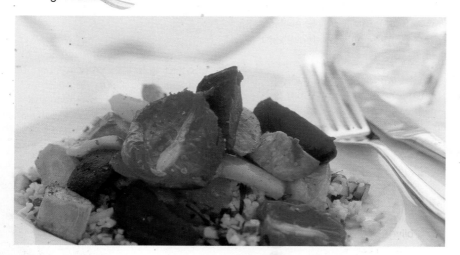

Roasted vegetables

2 large or 4 small uncooked beetroot, peeled and cut into quarters or chunks

2 large or 4 small carrots, peeled and cut into chunks

2 onions, peeled and cut into wedges

2 sweet potatoes, peeled and cut into chunks

4 plum tomatoes, halved

2 yellow peppers, de-seeded and halved

Extra virgin olive oil

Paprika

Low sodium salt

Black pepper

Bulghur wheat salad

110g/4 oz bulghur wheat

1 tomato, peeled, de-seeded and finely chopped

$1/2$ cucumber, core removed and flesh chopped finely

2 tbsp fresh chopped mint

2 tbsp fresh chopped parsley

Juice of 1 lemon

4 spring onions, trimmed and finely chopped

Extra virgin olive oil

Low sodium salt

Black pepper

Low fat live natural yoghurt to serve

Method

1   Lay the vegetables in roasting trays, drizzle with olive oil and sprinkle with the paprika and seasonings.

2   Roast in a hot oven at GM6/200C until tender. This will take about half an hour, depending on how large the vegetable chunks are.

3   Put peppers in a plastic bag, seal and allow to cool. This will allow the skins to slip off more easily later.

4   Whilst they are in the oven make the cracked wheat salad: Soak the wheat or lightly cook according to instructions on the packet.

5   Toss all the salad ingredients together, dress with the lemon juice and olive oil and season with a little low sodium salt and pepper.

6   Skin the roasted peppers and cut into quarters. Arrange the warm roasted vegetables on four plates, on a bed of the bulghur wheat salad and top with a teaspoon of live natural yoghurt and a pinch of paprika.

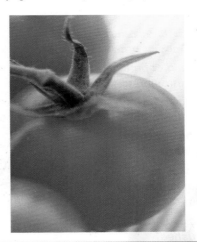

DR CLAYTON SAYS:

There is a growing body of evidence to suggest that Western diets contain too much protein from animal sources. **Bulghur wheat** is a whole-grain low-fat protein source that is high in dietary fibre, plus calcium and B complex vitamins.

Meanwhile the vegetables contribute a range of vitamins, minerals, flavonoids and carotenoids. **Beetroot** is rich in folate and potassium. **Carrots** and **sweet potatoes** are rich in beta-carotene, which is a precursor in the body for Vitamin A. **Yellow peppers** contain flavonoids.

Onions and **spring onions** are rich in quercitin, which neutralises free radicals, and pre-biotic fibre that encourages bowel health.

Tomatoes are rich in Vitamin C as well as containing the carotenoid lycopene, which may be particularly useful in protecting against prostate cancer.

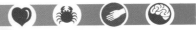

Shrimp stir fry

Serves 4

Time Guide
Preparation: 10 mins
Cooking time: 5 mins

250g/8oz rice noodles

450g/1lb frozen raw shrimps or prawns

1 head of broccoli, cut into florets

200g/7oz beansprouts

250g/8oz baby spinach

2 small leeks, trimmed and cut into diagonal strips

2 cloves garlic, crushed

2.5cm/1 inch piece root ginger, peeled and grated

1 tbsp groundnut oil

1 bunch spring onions, trimmed and chopped

1 tbsp sesame seeds

3 tbsp soy sauce

1/2 glass white wine

2 tbsp honey

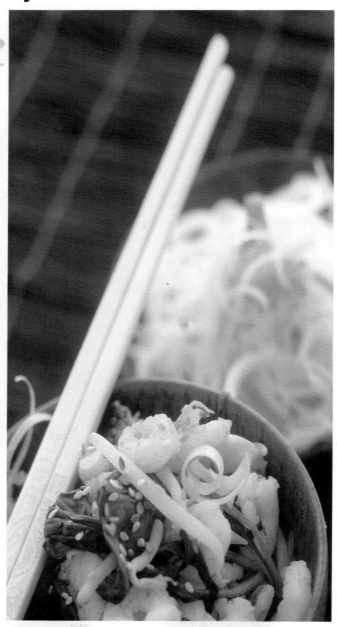

Method

1. In a wok heat the oil and, when hot, add the broccoli, ginger, leeks, garlic and shrimps, three quarters of the spring onions, the beansprouts and baby spinach. Stir fry for 2-3 minutes.

2. In the meantime soak the rice noodles as prescribed on the packet.

3. Mix together the soy sauce, honey and white wine and add to the wok. Continue to cook for a further minute.

4. Serve the noodles in individual bowls and top with the stir fry.

5. Sprinkle over the sesame seeds and the remaining spring onions.

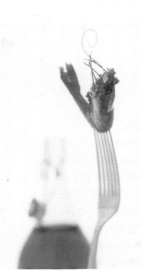

DR CLAYTON SAYS:

Quick, delicious and very nutritious.

Shrimps and **prawns** (especially fresh water ones) contain betaine, a methyl group donor which can reduce levels of the toxic metabolite homocysteine, thereby reducing the risk of heart attacks and Alzheimer's.

Both **spinach** and **broccoli** are good sources of Vitamin K, essential for healthy bones; lutein, which protects the eyes; and Vitamin C, which may help to prevent cancers; as well as dietary fibre.

Spring onions and **leeks** contain the flavonoid quercitin, which has anti-inflammatory and cardio-protective properties. They also contain prebiotic fibres, other dietary fibre, and some of the same cholesterol-reducing and anti-cancer sulphur compounds that are found in **garlic**.

Ginger provides ginger flavonoids which have marked anti-inflammatory properties and are particularly useful to sufferers from arthritis. These flavonoids are also probably cardio-protective.

Beansprouts are a good source of B vitamins and dietary fibre, with some Vitamin C.

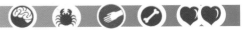

Baked stuffed mackerel with leek and lentils

Serves 2

Time Guide
Preparation: 15 mins
Cooking time: 45 mins

2 mackerel, cleaned and fins removed

55g/2oz feta cheese, cut into small cubes

2 tsp chopped fresh thyme

4 sundried tomatoes, very finely chopped

A little lemon juice

Lentils

55g/2oz puy lentils

1 glass red wine

1 glass water (100ml)

1 onion, very finely chopped

1 clove garlic, very finely chopped

Leeks

1 large leek, trimmed, cleaned and cut in half, each piece tied together around the 'waist' with some poultry string

1/2 pint vegetable stock

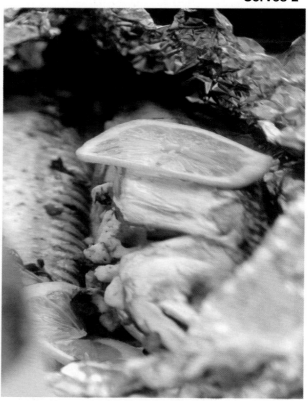

Method

1   Mix together the cubed feta, sundried tomatoes and fresh thyme with a little olive oil. Then stuff the cavities of the fish.

2   Place the fish in a roasting tray, sprinkle with a little more olive oil and lemon juice and season with black pepper. (The sundried tomatoes and feta are quite salty so you should not need salt.)

3   In a separate pan sweat the onion and garlic gently in a little olive oil until transparent and soft.

4 Add the rinsed puy lentils, pour over the red wine and water and bring up to simmering point. Let the lentils cook until tender. If drying out before tender, add a little of the leek stock.

5 In a separate pan heat the vegetable stock, drop in the tied-up leeks and allow to gently poach for about 10-15 minutes. When tender, drain and remove the string.

6 Cover the filled mackerel with tin foil and put in a pre heated oven (GM6/200C) for about 15 minutes, or until cooked through and the filling hot.

7 Serve the mackerel with the lentils and poached leek.

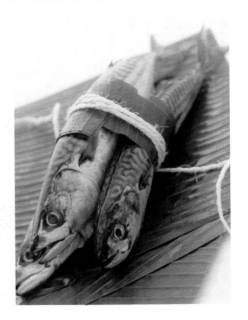

DR CLAYTON SAYS:

This ingredients in this recipe can help protect against many of the major degenerative diseases.

Mackerel is an oily fish, which is rich in Omega 3 to protect against coronary artery disease. It is also high in Vitamin D, essential for calcium absorption in the body, Vitamin B12, and minerals such as iodine.

Red wine contains flavonoids with powerful anti-cancer, anti-clotting and cardio-protective properties.

Thyme and garlic are powerful anti-oxidants. Leeks contain the flavonoid quercitin that neutralises free radical action in the body. The pre-biotic content encourages a healthy bowel and digestive system.

Puy lentils are an excellent, low fat source of protein and dietary fibre. They also provide a good source of minerals and B vitamins and may help to control blood sugar and lower blood cholesterol. Feta cheese is rich in calcium.

Vegetable cassoulet

Serves 4

Time Guide

Preparation: 25 mins

Cooking time: 1 hour

2 x 400g/14oz cans
haricot beans

1 x 400g/14oz can soya
beans

1 onion, sliced

2 cloves garlic, crushed

Extra virgin olive oil

2 carrots, peeled and
cut into dice

1 large or 2 small sticks
of celery, diced

1 glass red wine

$1/2$ tbsp fresh oregano

$1/2$ tbsp fresh thyme

$1/2$ tbsp fresh parsley

1 x 400g/14oz tin
chopped tomatoes

2 courgettes, cut into
dice

330g/12oz spinach

12 sundried tomatoes,
cut into strips (reserve
some of the olive oil)

Low sodium salt

Black pepper

Bay leaf

3 slices wholemeal
bread, made into
crumbs

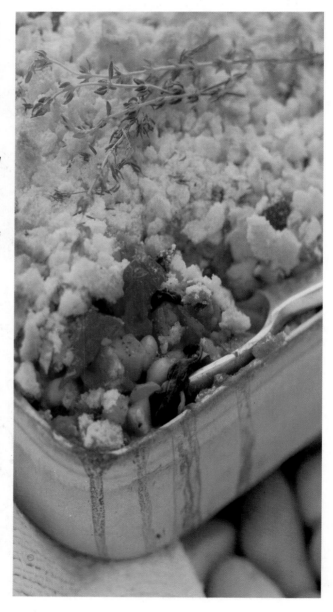

Method

1 In a large heavy based pan, sweat the sliced onion in the olive oil and add the garlic, carrots, celery and red wine. Allow to cook for a couple of minutes.

2 Add the tinned beans and tin of chopped tomatoes, courgettes, sundried tomatoes, spinach and herbs. Season with a little low sodium salt and black pepper.

3 If the mixture looks at all dry, add a few tablespoons of water.

4 Transfer all the ingredients to an ovenproof dish and cover with a layer of breadcrumbs, drizzle over some of the reserved oil from the sundried tomatoes.

5 Bake in a preheated oven, GM5/190C for about 30 minutes until the breadcrumbs are golden. Serve immediately.

DR CLAYTON SAYS:

A substantial and tasty vegetarian dish high in a range of important micro-nutrients.

Soya beans are high in protein with a healthy balance of amino acids. They contain a balance of soluble and insoluble fibre to promote a healthy digestive system and protect against bowel cancers. They are also a rich source of genistein, an isoflavone that not only inhibits the growth of cancer cells, but can also force them to revert to normal.

Haricot beans also have good fibre and protein content. They are a good source of B vitamins and can help to control blood sugar levels.

Onions are rich in the flavonoid quercitin, which can help to neutralise free radicals in the body.

Garlic contains anti-oxidants which can protect the cholesterol in the arteries from oxidising and are, therefore, cardio-protective.

Red wine contains flavonoids with powerful anti-cancer, anti-clotting and cardio-protective properties. **Tomatoes** are a source of Vitamin C as well as containing the carotenoid lycopene, which has anti-cancer properties.

Spinach is a good source of Vitamin K, lutein and beta-carotene; as are **carrots**. Lutein and beta carotene protect the skin and eyes and may also have cardio- and cancer-protecting properties.

Sardines baked in tomato sauce

Serves 2

4-6 sardines,
depending on size,
cleaned and gutted

Small handful fresh
basil leaves

Tomato sauce

1 carrot, peeled and
finely chopped

1 stick celery, finely
chopped

1 small onion,
peeled and finely
chopped

1 clove of garlic,
peeled and finely
chopped

2 tbsp extra virgin
olive oil

1x 400g/14oz tin
chopped tomatoes

1 tbsp tomato puree

Small glass red wine

8-10 olives

1 tbsp capers

Low sodium salt

Freshly ground
black pepper

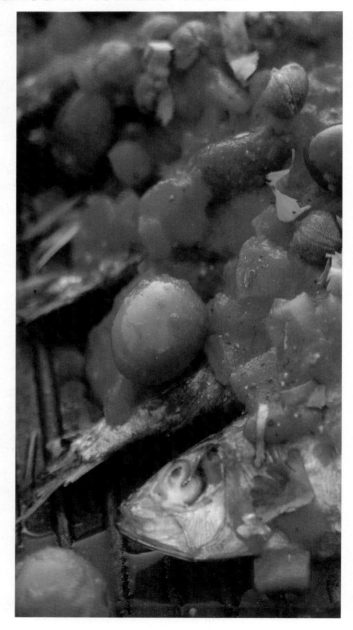

Method

1 To make the sauce, sweat the first five ingredients together until soft but not coloured. Then add the tinned tomatoes, tomato puree and red wine. Season to taste with low sodium salt and pepper. Add the olives and capers and stir well.

2 Clean the sardines, arrange in an ovenproof dish and pour over the tomato sauce.

3 Bake in a preheated oven GM4/180C for about 20 minutes until heated through.

3 Garnish with torn basil leaves and serve immediately with a green salad of watercress, cucumber, onion dressed with olive oil and lemon juice and boiled new potatoes.

Time Guide

Preparation: 15 mins
Cooking time: 20 mins

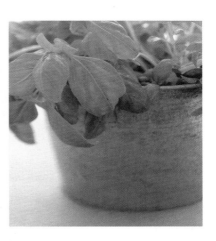

DR CLAYTON SAYS:

Another power-packed recipe full of micro-nutrients offering broad spectrum protection against many of the main degenerative diseases.

Sardines are an excellent source of Omega 3, the fish oil providing protection against heart disease.

The mono-unsaturated fatty acids (MUFAs) in **olives** (as in olive oil, of course, too) also protect the heart, and lower blood pressure and cholesterol.

Red wine contains a group of flavonoids that protect the heart and blood vessels as well as helping maintain the elasticity of the skin.

Tomatoes are a good source of both Vitamin C and lycopene, an anti-cancer carotenoid, which may be effective in protecting against prostate cancer.

Wild salmon oatcakes with caper sauce

Serves 2-3 (makes 8 small or 6 large fishcakes)

Salmon oatcakes

1 x 400g/14oz tin wild red salmon

85g/3oz oats

80ml/2 fl oz skimmed milk

1 free range egg

2 tbsp chopped dill or chervil

Low sodium salt

Black pepper

Extra virgin olive oil

6 tbsp fresh breadcrumbs

Caper sauce

Small carton of low fat, live natural yoghurt

1 pickled gherkin, chopped very finely

2 tbsp capers, chopped very finely

Low sodium salt

Black pepper

1 tsp chopped chives

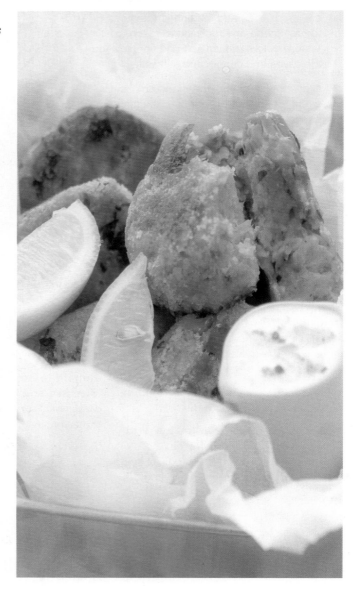

Method

1   Mix sauce ingredients together, season and chill.

2   Combine together all salmon ingredients except the olive oil and breadcrumbs.

3   Shape the cakes into rounds about 2 cm($3/4$ inch) thick and roll in the breadcrumbs.

4   Heat a little olive oil in a non-stick frying pan and brown each fishcake for about 3-4 minutes each side over a medium heat.

5   Serve with the sauce and a wedge of lemon, with boiled new potatoes and green beans.

Time Guide

Preparation: 15-20 mins

Cooking time: 10 mins

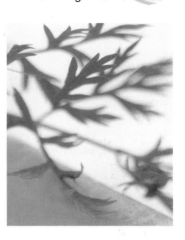

DR CLAYTON SAYS:

The ingredients in this recipe have strongly cardio-protective properties.

Salmon contains significant levels of the valuable cardio-protective Omega 3 oils; **oats** have been shown to lower total blood cholesterol; **olive oil** lowers the level of 'bad' LDL cholesterol; and **eggs** increase the level of 'good' HDL cholesterol.

The carotenoids in the **eggs** and **salmon** (the deeper the colour, the higher the carotenoid content), and the flavonoids in **olive oil** have anti-cancer and anti-oxidant properties.

The live natural **yoghurt** contains pro-biotic bacteria that help protect against gastro-intestinal infection.

Oats contain beta glucans, an excellent pre-biotic that protects the lower bowel and liver.

If you use **wholemeal bread** for the breadcrumbs, you will be adding dietary fibre, as well as B vitamins, calcium and magnesium.

Spinach, pear and feta cheese pasta salad

Serves 4

450g/1lb penne or fusilli pasta shapes, cooked and cooled

375g/12oz baby spinach leaves

2 ripe pears, skin on and sliced

2 yellow peppers, deseeded and sliced

Half a cucumber, sliced thinly

120g/4$^1/_2$ oz feta cheese

2 tbsp fresh parsley, chopped

Dressing

100ml extra virgin olive oil

30ml balsamic vinegar

1 generous tbsp runny honey

Low sodium salt and freshly ground black pepper

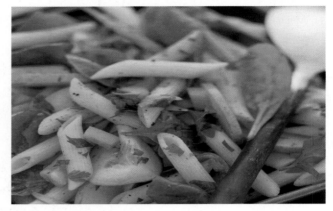

Method

1   For the dressing, mix together the extra virgin olive oil, balsamic vinegar, honey, low sodium salt and black pepper.

2   Then mix together the first six ingredients in a roomy bowl. Pour over a little of the dressing and toss well. Sprinkle with the chopped parsley.

DR CLAYTON SAYS:

Pasta is a healthy low fat source of both protein and complex carbohydrate, with an intermediate glycemic index.

Spinach contains Vitamin K, lutein, beta carotene and Vitamin C (anti-oxidants), and potassium which can help lower blood pressure, as well as folate. Yellow peppers are another good source of Vitamin C.

Pears are a good source of dietary fibre, essential for a healthy digestive system as well as being a good source of potassium and Vitamin C. Pear skin contains immuno-stimulants similar to those in Echinacea and shiitake mushrooms.

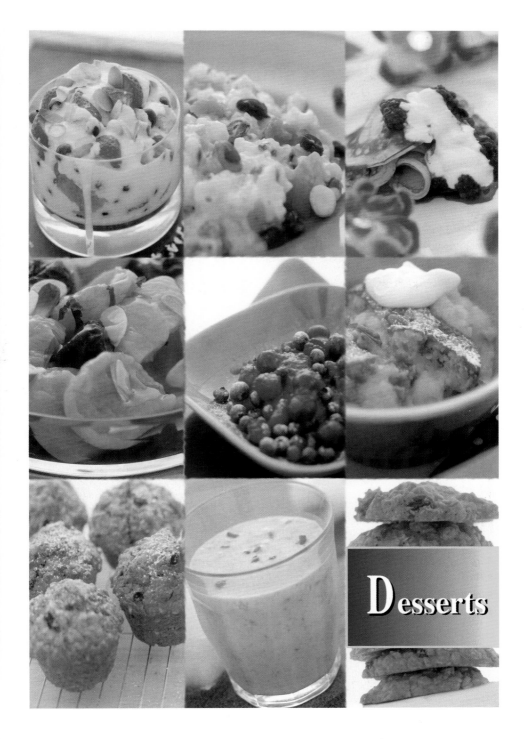

Desserts

"I can't believe it's not trifle"

Serves 4

*570ml/1 pint live
natural yoghurt*

*1 x 200g/7oz tub low
fat crème fraiche*

*2 large mangoes,
stone and skin
removed, chopped
or 250g/9oz tinned
mango pulp*

*1 x 225g/8oz punnet
blueberries, washed*

450g/1lb strawberries

*30g/1oz chopped
almonds*

Sponge

3 free range eggs

*85g/3oz golden
caster sugar*

1 1/2 tbsp warm water

*85g/3oz plain flour,
sifted*

*Pinch low sodium
salt*

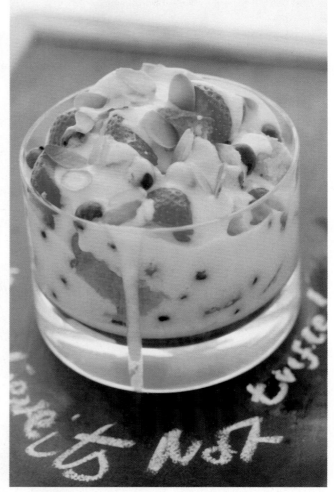

Method

First make the sponge:

1   Set the oven at GM4/180C. Prepare a cake
    tin,18cm/7 inch or 20cm/8 inch in diameter, by
    lining with parchment.

2　Place eggs and sugar in a bowl and using an electric beater, whisk until light, thick and fluffy, and then add the water.

3　Sift the flour and salt and, with a large metal spoon, fold into the mixture, being careful not to beat out any air.

4　Turn the mixture into the prepared tin and bake in the middle of the oven for about 25-30 minutes. You will be able to tell whether the cake is cooked, as it will shrink away from the sides. If you use the larger cake tin, it will cook slightly quicker.

5　Cool on a wire rack. When ready to use cut into pieces.

To assemble the trifle:

1　Mix together the yoghurt and the crème fraiche.

2　In a blender liquidise the mango or measure out the tinned pulp and fold this into the yoghurt mixture.

3　Put a layer of yoghurt mix in the bottom of a bowl and top with pieces of the sponge. Moisten if necessary with a little apple juice, then add a layer of blueberries and strawberries.

4　Continue to layer up finishing with a layer of yoghurt. Sprinkle the top with the toasted, flaked almonds and decorate with whole strawberries. Refrigerate for 2 hours and serve.

DR CLAYTON SAYS:

It's difficult to believe that this super dessert is also nutritious. But it is because the 'nasties' in a traditional trifle have been substituted by nutritious 'goodies'.

Eggs are unusual in that they contain saturated fats, but in the form of phospholipids which increase good HDL cholesterol levels. Vitamin D is also found in eggs and is essential for the uptake and distribution of calcium in the body.

Natural live yoghurt contains pro-biotics ('healthy' bacteria), some of which can help reduce the risk of food poisoning. Yoghurt and crème fraiche are also rich in calcium essential for bone growth and repair.

Mangoes, strawberries and blueberries are all rich sources of the anti-oxidant Vitamin C. Mangoes have the added advantage of being high in beta carotene, which the body converts to Vitamin A, which is vital to maintain healthy vision. Blueberries also contain high levels of flavonoids linked to increased protection against heart disease and various cancers.

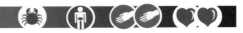

Spiced pears with a pair of sauces

Time Guide

Serves 4

Preparation: 15 mins

Cooking time: 40 mins

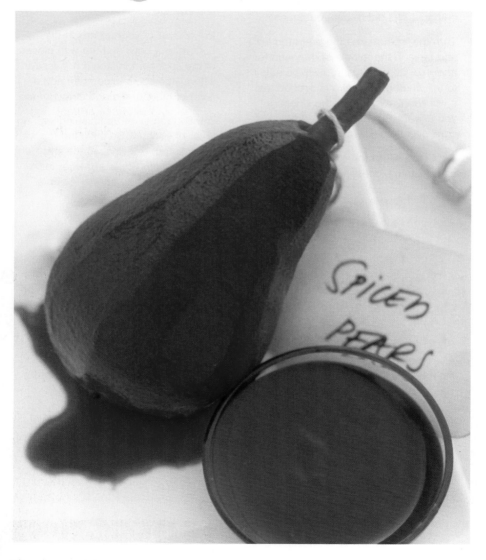

Method

1. The pears need to be stood up in a pan just big enough to accommodate them. Pour over the red wine, water, sugar and cinnamon stick.

2. Poach until soft, about 20 minutes, depending on the ripeness of the fruit.

3. Remove from the liquor and put aside to cool. Remove the cinnamon stick and reduce down the liquid to a thick sauce. Remove from heat and allow to cool.

4. In a bain-marie over a pan of gently simmering water melt the chocolate with the small knob of butter.

5. Serve the pears, whole or sliced and fanned with two pools of sauces (chocolate and red wine) one either side of the pear.

6. If desired dot crème fraiche in the chocolate sauce and draw a cocktail stick through it to feather it.

4 pears, peeled and left whole

290ml/$^1/_2$ pint red wine (preferably Cabernet Sauvignon)

Enough water to cover

30g/1oz caster sugar

1 cinnamon stick

100g dark chocolate (70% cocoa solids)

Small knob of butter

2 tbsp low fat crème fraiche

DR CLAYTON SAYS:

Pears are a good source of dietary fibre, the anti-oxidant Vitamin C and potassium.

Red wine is another potent anti-oxidant that prevents oxidative damage in the walls of blood vessels and thus protects against heart disease. It also contains a flavonoid resveratrol, which raises good HDL cholesterol and reduces platelet stickiness. These flavonoids can also form a protective shield around collagen and elastin fibres, which give skin its firmness and texture and protect them against enzymes which break down these fibres and against free radical damage.

Dark chocolate with a high percentage of cocoa solids (70% and above) is a good source of anti-oxidants. The darker the chocolate, the higher the cocoa solids content, the more flavonoid it contains and the healthier it is. Milk chocolate, on the other hand, cannot be regarded as a health food!

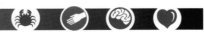

Crimson compote

Serves 4

Time Guide
Preparation: 15 mins
Chilling time: 1 hour

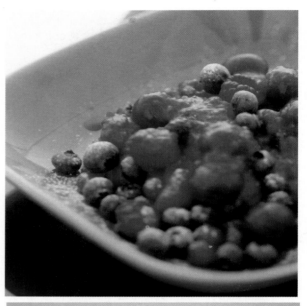

450g/1lb strawberries

225g/8oz black/red cherries

225g/8oz raspberries

225g/8oz redcurrants

225g/8oz blueberries

Golden caster sugar to taste

100ml red grape juice

Low fat crème fraiche/natural live yoghurt to serve

Method

1   Liquidise half the strawberries with the red grape juice.

2   Taste and add a little sugar if necessary.

3   Pour this puree over the remaining washed fruit and chill until ready to serve.

DR CLAYTON SAYS:

For me, this recipe represents the ideal way to step up my intake of anti-oxidants and pro-biotics.

Strawberries, cherries, raspberries, redcurrants, blueberries are all rich in the anti-oxidant Vitamin C and flavonoids which help prevent oxidative damage. Darker fruits contain more flavonoids.

Red grape juice is rich in flavonoids (although not as rich as red wine) which protect against heart and blood vessel damage by free radicals in the body. Like red wine, it has anti-clotting effects.

Natural low fat **live yoghurt** contains pro-biotics, 'healthy bacteria' which can help to promote a healthy bowel. Yoghurt and crème fraiche are both rich in calcium, essential for bone growth and repair.

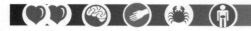

Oat and carrot muffins

Makes 10

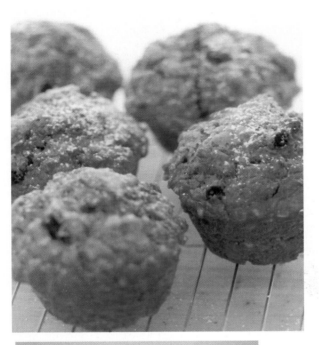

Time Guide
Preparation: 15 mins
Cooking time: 20 mins

170g/6oz plain flour

85g/3oz oats

1 medium carrot, peeled and grated

75g/2$\frac{1}{2}$oz raisins

75g/2$\frac{1}{2}$oz dark brown sugar

1 tbsp baking powder

1 tsp ground cinnamon

$\frac{1}{2}$ tsp bicarbonate of soda

3 tbsp skimmed milk

2 free range eggs, lightly beaten

50ml sunflower oil

1 tsp vanilla essence

Icing sugar to dust

DR CLAYTON SAYS:

Oats are rich in pre-biotics to promote a healthy gut, and protect against bowel cancers and food poisoning. They are also useful for those trying to lose weight as they give a feeling of fullness and may suppress appetite. The soluble fibre in oats is also useful in lowering 'bad' LDL cholesterol levels and therefore is beneficial to the heart and circulatory system.

Carrots are a good source of beta-carotene, which the body converts to Vitamin A to maintain healthy vision.

Method

1 Line muffin cups with paper cases.

2 Mix together all the ingredients except the icing sugar.

3 Divide between the 10 muffin cups and bake in a preheated oven at GM5/190C for about 20 minutes.

4 Allow to cool on a rack and lightly dust with icing sugar. Serve when slightly cooled.

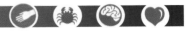

Mulled wine jelly

Serves 4

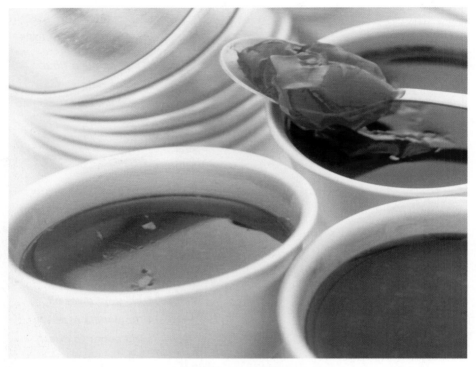

Time Guide

Preparation: 20 mins
Cooking time: 15 mins
Chilling time: 2-3 hours

290ml/¹/₂ pint Cabernet Sauvignon red wine (or unsweetened red grape juice)

Cinnamon stick

2 whole cloves

60ml/4 tbsp freshly squeezed orange juice (use lemon juice if using grape juice as it is sweeter)

60ml/4 tbsp sugar syrup, infused with cinnamon stick

Gelatine or agar-agar (vegetarian alternative) – amount as per manufacturer's instructions to set ³/₄ pint of liquid

Black cherries, to serve

Low fat crème fraiche, to serve

Method

1 Make a sugar syrup using 5oz sugar to 290ml/$\frac{1}{2}$ pint water by dissolving the sugar in the water and boiling for 4-5 minutes.

2 Heat the wine in a pan with the cinnamon stick and cloves and bring to a simmer. Remove from the heat and allow to infuse for about 20 minutes.

3 Put the orange juice and sugar syrup into another pan and sprinkle over the gelatine (always in that order, or the gelatine may go lumpy).

4 Heat the gelatine on a very low heat until it has dissolved. (Do not allow it to overheat as it will become stringy and will not set.)

5 Remove the cinnamon stick and cloves from the infused wine and add the gelatine mixture to it. Stir gently to mix thoroughly and pour into a wet bowl or mould.

6 Leave in the fridge to set for at least 2-3 hours before turning out.

7 Serve with a black cherry compote made with fresh or tinned cherries in natural juice, and crème fraiche.

DR CLAYTON SAYS:

Red wine (particularly Cabernet Sauvignon) contains potent anti-oxidant flavonoids that prevents oxidative damage in the walls of blood vessels and thus protect against heart disease. Similar flavonoids are reported to help varicose veins and oedema of the lower limbs. It also contains a flavonoid resveratrol, which raises good HDL cholesterol and reduces platelet stickiness.

These flavonoids also form a protective shield around collagen and elastin fibres, which give skin its firmness and texture and protect them against enzymes which break down these fibres and against free radical damage.

Black cherries and **orange juice** are both good sources of Vitamin C, another powerful anti-oxidant to protect against the degenerative diseases. **Cherries** also contain flavonoids for additional protective effects.

Low fat **crème fraiche** is a good source of calcium essential for the growth and repair of bones.

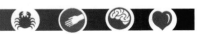

Fruit and nut rice pudding

Serves 4

Time Guide
Preparation: 5 mins
Cooking time: 40 mins

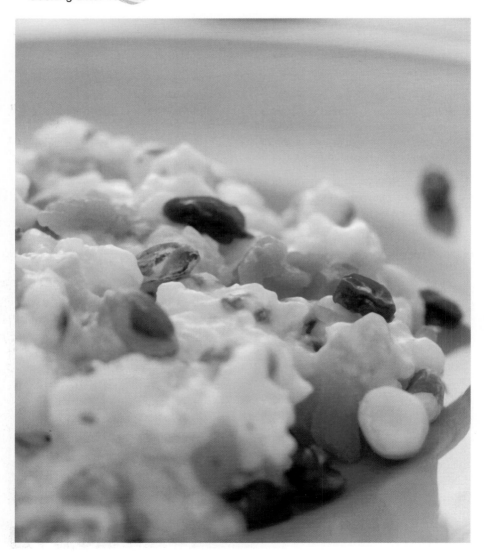

Method

1 In a pan heat the rice and milk together, bring up to the boil and turn down to a simmer. Cook gently for 30 minutes, keeping an eye on the mixture.

2 Add the nuts, apricots, raisins, cardamom pods and sugar and cook for a further 10 minutes, adding a little more milk if the mixture is starting to look a little dry.

3 Serve immediately. Or cool, refrigerate and reheat when required.

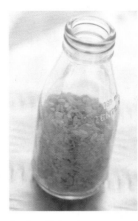

55g/2oz pudding rice

570ml/1 pint skimmed milk

1^1/$_2$ tbsp golden caster sugar

5 cardamom pods, slit open and seeds crushed in a pestle and mortar

30g/1oz shelled Brazil nuts, roughly chopped

55g/2oz shelled pistachio nuts, roughly chopped

6 dried apricots, chopped

55g/2oz raisins

DR CLAYTON SAYS:

The addition of **dried fruit** and **nuts** makes this rice pudding a good provider of flavonoids, anti-oxidants and minerals, as well as giving it much more appeal.

Rice is a useful source of complex carbohydrates, used as fuel for the body. Use **skimmed milk** for the benefit of a high calcium content without excess saturated fat.

Nuts are an excellent source of Vitamin E, an anti-oxidant essential for a healthy heart as well as B vitamins. They also provide a useful source of protein, particularly in a vegetarian diet. **Brazil nuts** also contain Omega 6 PUFAs and the anti-cancer mineral selenium.

Dried apricots are a rich source of beta carotene and fibre, and are also rich in iron and potassium, which has been associated with a decrease in blood pressure. **Raisins** are high in flavonoids that protect the heart from oxidative damage in the blood vessel walls.

Oat and raisin cookies

Makes 12

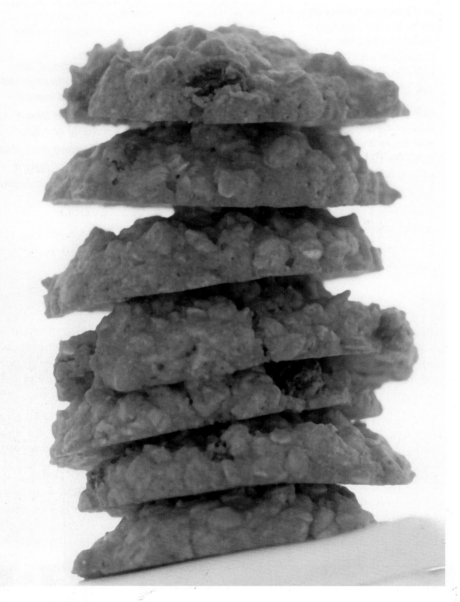

Method

1   In a bowl mix together the dark brown sugar with the butter and beat (with an electric whisk) until fluffy and soft. Add the maple syrup and whisk until incorporated.

2   Add the egg whites and the other remaining ingredients and mix well with a wooden spoon.

3   Spoon onto a baking sheet lined with baking parchment, and flatten slightly with the back of a spoon, leaving at least 1cm/$^1/_2$ inch between each cookie to allow for spreading.

4   Bake in a preheated oven GM5/190C for about 12-15 minutes.

5   Allow to cool, then store in an airtight container.

6   The raisins could be substituted for chopped very dark chocolate pieces (70% cocoa solids).

Time Guide

Preparation: 15-20 mins
Cooking time: 15 mins

85g/3oz dark brown soft sugar

70g/2$^1/_2$oz butter

100ml/4fl oz maple syrup

2 egg whites, lightly beaten

1 tsp vanilla essence

200g/7oz oats

30g/1oz raisins

125g/4$^1/_2$oz plain flour

$^1/_2$ tsp bicarbonate of soda

$^1/_2$ tsp low sodium salt

DR CLAYTON SAYS:

The ideal 'tastes good, does you good' snack.

Oats are rich in pre-biotics to promote a healthy gut, and protect against bowel cancers and food poisoning. They may be useful for those who are trying to lose weight as they give a feeling of fullness and may suppress appetite. The soluble fibre in oats is also useful in lowering 'bad' LDL cholesterol levels and therefore is beneficial to the heart and circulatory system.

Raisins are high in flavonoids that protect the heart from oxidative damage in the blood vessel walls. A lower sodium, higher potassium and magnesium salt alternative is useful in helping to lower blood pressure.

Apple, pecan and ginger pudding
Serves 4

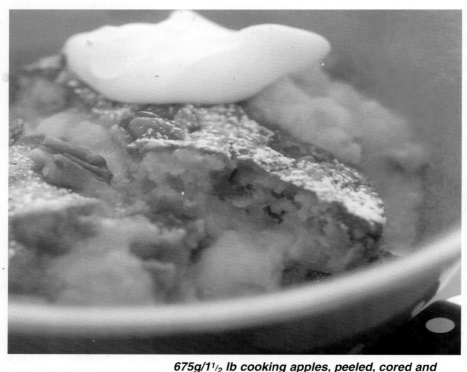

Time Guide

Preparation: 25 mins
Cooking time: 40 mins

675g/1¹/₂ lb cooking apples, peeled, cored and cut into chunks

140g/5oz caster sugar

120ml/¹/₄ pt water

30g/1oz butter

1 free range egg, beaten

55g/2oz self-raising flour

Pinch low sodium salt

3 pieces stem ginger, finely chopped

2 tbsp ginger syrup

12 pecan halves, roughly chopped

A dash of skimmed milk if necessary

A little sunflower oil for greasing

Method

1   Place the apples, 110g/4oz of sugar and the water in a pan and stew until the apple is tender.

2   In a bowl and with an electric whisk beat together the butter and remaining 30g/1oz sugar until fluffy. Add the beaten egg slowly, with a teaspoon of flour if it looks as if it might start to curdle. Add a pinch of low sodium salt.

3   Fold in the remaining flour, then add the ginger syrup and stir in the chopped ginger and pecans.

4   Put the apple in the base of a greased pudding basin and top with the sponge mixture.

5   Bake for about 25-30 mins at GM5/190C.

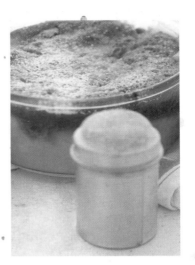

DR CLAYTON SAYS:

A variation on the traditional Eve's Pudding, this dessert adds the anti-cancer and anti-inflammatory benefits of **ginger** and **pecan nuts** to the cardio-protective qualities of **apples**.

Apples are rich in the flavonoid quercitin (also found in onions and leeks) which may be one of the most cardio-protective substances yet discovered. It protects the lipids in blood from oxidising and therefore protects the heart. Apples are also rich in chromium, which may help to regulate sugar cravings and insulin levels in the body.

Egg yolks, while they contain saturated fats, are rich in phospho-lipids, which actually raise good HDL cholesterol. In addition they are a source of carotenoids and of Vitamin D, vital in the absorption and distribution of calcium in the body.

Ginger, as well as being a powerful anti-oxidant to give a wide ranging protection against the major degenerative diseases, is also an effective anti-inflammatory useful to sufferers of conditions such as arthritis.

Pecans are a good source of protein and provide Vitamin E and the B vitamins.

Strawberry and ginger sorbet

Serves 4

Time Guide
Preparation: 30 mins
Chilling time: 1-2 hours

170g/6oz golden caster sugar

570ml/1 pint water

4 tbsp stem ginger syrup

Juice of half a lemon

340g/12oz fresh/frozen/ tinned and drained strawberries

4 pieces of stem ginger, very finely chopped

2 egg whites

4 fresh strawberries to decorate (optional)

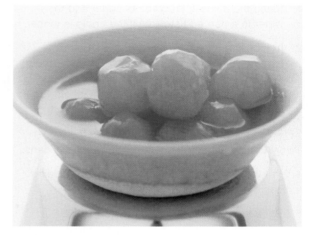

DR CLAYTON SAYS:

A delicious summer dessert which is rich in anti-oxidants.

Ginger, as well as being a powerful anti-oxidant to give a wide ranging protection against the major degenerative diseases, is also an effective anti-inflammatory useful to sufferers of conditions such as arthritis.

Strawberries are a good source of Vitamin C and have some flavonoids.

Method

1   Place the sugar and water together in a thick-bottomed saucepan. Dissolve over a gentle heat, and when clear, boil gently for 5 minutes to give a syrup. Add the ginger syrup and lemon juice to this.

2   Liquidise the strawberries to a pulp and add the syrup. Put in a freezer-proof container, and transfer to the freezer for 1 to 2 hours or until the mixture is beginning to solidify. Put the frozen mixture into a food processor, and mix until soft. Whisk the egg white and pour into the food processor with the motor still running. Fold in the chopped ginger and return to freezer until solid.

3   Before serving allow to come to room temperature for about 10 minutes.

Warning: Not suitable for pregnant women, who should not eat raw eggs.

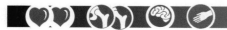

Banana and strawberry smoothie

Serves 2

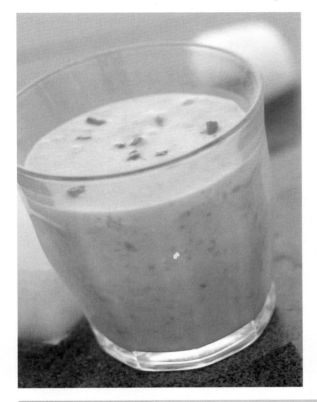

Time Guide
Preparation: 3 mins

12 ripe strawberries

1 large ripe banana

1 small carton low fat, live natural yoghurt

A couple of tablespoons of skimmed milk if necessary to 'let down'

4 ice cubes

Runny honey (to taste)

Method

1   Place all of the above in a blender and process to a thick shake-like drink.

2   Serve immediately.

DR CLAYTON SAYS:

Try this 'smoothie' as a dessert or a nutritious and filling 'snack drink' between meals.

The banana contributes pre-biotic fibre; and live yoghurt is a pro-biotic; together they maintain the healthy bacteria in the gut, and promote general health in the gut and bowel.

Strawberries are a rich source of Vitamin C, and contain some anti-cancer flavonoids.

Bananas are also high in potassium, which has been reported to reduce blood pressure. Low fat yoghurt and skimmed milk contribute calcium, without the negatives of high saturated fat.

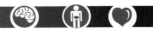

Sweet pancakes with fruit compote

Time Guide

Serves 4 (makes 8 pancakes)

Preparation: 5 mins
Cooking time: 15 mins

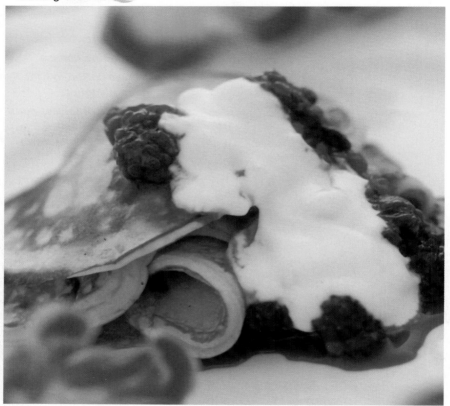

Pancakes

450g/1lb carton low fat fromage frais

130g/4¹/₂ oz self-raising flour

2 free range eggs, beaten

110g/4oz golden caster sugar

A few drops of vanilla essence

Compote

400g/14oz blackcurrants, blackberries, raspberries or other soft fruit (fresh or frozen)

Golden caster sugar – to taste

Little lemon juice

To serve

Low fat crème fraiche or live natural yoghurt

Method

1   First make the batter by mixing together the fromage frais, flour, eggs and vanilla essence. Finally stir in the sugar.

2   Fry spoonfuls of the batter in a few drops of sunflower oil in a good non-stick pan.

3   While you are frying the batches of pancakes, lightly cook the compote. Put the fruit and a tablespoon or two of water in a pan and heat through until the fruit starts to form a jam-like mixture. Season with caster sugar and a little lemon juice if desired.

4   Keep each batch of pancakes warm, and when all are ready serve two per person with some of the warm fruit compote and crème fraiche or live natural yoghurt.

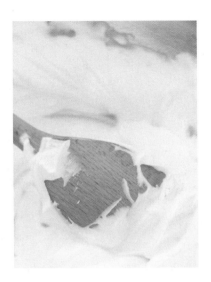

DR CLAYTON SAYS:

Blackcurrants are among the best sources of a valuable flavonoid group linked to good protection against heart disease and various cancers, and which can reduce the signs of ageing by preventing the breakdown of collagen and elastin in the skin. They also contain high levels of Vitamin C.

Blackberries, raspberries and strawberries also contain high levels of Vitamin C, but have a lower flavonoid content than blackcurrants.

Egg yolks are rich in phospholipids, which raise 'good' HDL cholesterol.

They also contain Vitamin D, vital in the absorption and distribution of calcium in the body.

Whenever you can, top your desserts with low fat live yoghurt, rather than any other milk product. It is a rich source of calcium (like other milk products), but has the added advantages of being low in saturated fat, and a pro-biotic, which maintains the healthy bacteria in the gut and promotes general health in the gut and bowel.

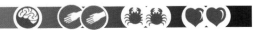

Dried fruit salad with honeyed green tea
Serves 4

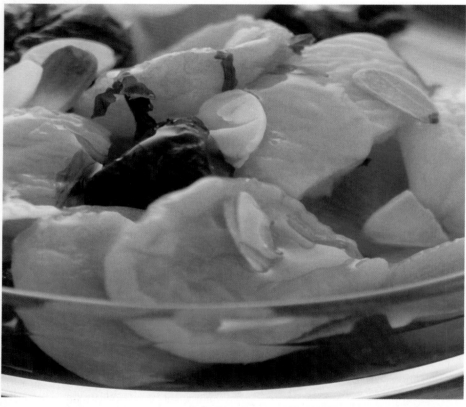

Time Guide

Preparation: 10 mins

Cooking time: 30 mins

Dried fruits – preferably the 'no need to soak' variety

> *100g/4oz dried apricots*
>
> *50g/2oz dried prunes*
>
> *100g/4oz dried pear slices*
>
> *100g/4oz dried apple slices/peaches*

850ml/1½ pints hot green tea

Runny honey

Toasted flaked almonds

Method

1   Make the tea and allow to brew for 2-3 minutes.

2   Soak the fruit salad in the strained hot tea for about 10 minutes then transfer to a pan and cook for about 20 minutes until tender (but not becoming mushy).

3   Remove fruit to a bowl with a slotted spoon.

4   Reduce down the tea liquor by about two-thirds. Taste and add honey as required to make a syrup.

5   Allow to cool and pour back over the fruit.

6   Serve scattered with toasted, flaked almonds.

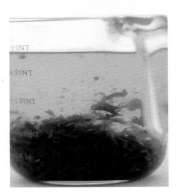

DR CLAYTON SAYS:

An ideal way of increasing micro-nutrient intake in the winter when fresh fruits are unavailable or expensive.

Dried fruits are an excellent source of dietary fibre, which is essential for a healthy gut. They are also rich in anti-oxidant vitamins and minerals that give a general protection against the major degenerative diseases. The drying process does not reduce micro-nutrient content appreciably.

Apricots are high in beta carotene and fibre, as well as iron and potassium, which has been associated with a decrease in blood pressure. **Prunes** have high levels of flavonoids.

Pears also contribute potassium.

Apples are rich in quercitin, a powerful cardio-protective flavonoid, and chromium, which may help the body to regulate sugar cravings and excess levels of insulin.

Green tea is high in flavonoids which are vital anti-oxidants important in preventing cancers and the other major degenerative diseases. Green tea has also been shown to be a good source of fluoride.

Almonds are a good source of protein and Vitamin E and B vitamins.

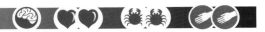

Muesli fruit crumble

Serves 4

Time Guide
Preparation: 10-15 mins
Cooking time: 25 mins

1kg/2lb ripe pears,
peeled, cored and diced

225g/¹/₂lb blackberries
(fresh or frozen)

A little water

Golden caster sugar

Topping

170g/6oz 'no added
sugar' muesli

3-4 tbsp honey

55g/2oz butter

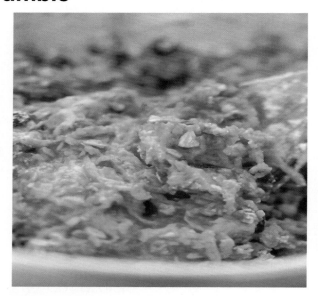

DR CLAYTON SAYS:

Using muesli instead of flour in a crumble gives the benefit of oats, dried fruit and nuts.

Oats have been shown to lower blood cholesterol, and they contain a pre-biotic which protects the lower bowel and liver.

Pears and **blackberries** are both high in Vitamin C, and blackberries also contain flavonoids for cancer and heart disease protection.

Raisins and **currants** are good sources of flavonoids, while most **nuts** provide the anti-oxidant Vitamin E.

Method

1   Put the fruit in an ovenproof dish and sprinkle with a little caster sugar, depending on how sweet the fruit is.

2   Mix together the muesli and butter with your fingers. Next add honey until loosely bound together. Spread on top of the fruit.

3   Bake in a pre-heated oven at GM4/180C for about 30-40 minutes. Check after about 20 minutes to see if the topping is becoming too brown. If it is, then loosely cover with foil and remove for the final 4-5 minutes to allow it to crisp up again.

4   Serve with yoghurt, crème fraiche or custard (made with fresh egg yolk, a little sugar, vanilla essence and skimmed milk).

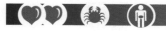

Index

Index

Acknowledgements

We acknowledge with thanks the contributions of the following who lent crockery and cutlery for the photography:

Robert Welch Designs Ltd, Chipping Campden, GL55 6DY

Trauffler, 100 East Rd, London N1 6AA

Divertimenti, Fulham Road, London SW3

Dudson, Scotia Rd, Tunstall, Stoke on Trent

Fired Earth, 117-119 Fulham Road, London, SW3 6RL

Also to Will Edridge for his assistance at the photographic shoot.

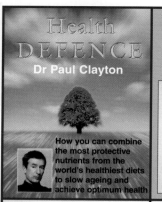